560-211

THE
FUNCTIONING
CYTOPLASM

THE FUNCTIONING CYTOPLASM

RUTH ELLEN BULGER
University of Maryland

JUDY MAY STRUM
University of California,
San Francisco Medical Center

PLENUM PRESS • NEW YORK AND LONDON

Library of Congress Cataloging in Publication Data

Bulger, Ruth Ellen.
    The functioning cytoplasm.

    Includes bibliographies.
    1. Cytology. 2. Cell physiology. I. Strum,
Judy May, joint author. II. Title. [DNLM: 1. Cyto-
logy. 2. Cytoplasm—Physiology. QH591 B933f 1973]
QH581.2.B84   574.8'7   73-7570
ISBN 0-306-30807-X

© 1974 Plenum Press, New York
A Division of Plenum Publishing Corporation
227 West 17th Street, New York, N.Y. 10011

United Kingdom edition published by Plenum Press, London
A Division of Plenum Publishing Company, Ltd.
4a Lower John Street, London, W1R 3PD, England

Printed in the United States of America

CONTENTS

PREFACE

This book was not written for contemporary scientists with a major interest in cell biology. Rather, it was prepared for the serious and inquiring student who may or may not have had an extensive background in the sciences but who is interested in exploring or reviewing in depth the current body of knowledge about cellular structure and function. We have tried to convey a sense of the expectant excitement that characterizes the modern-day cellular biologist and we regret any scientific jargon that may have crept into the text as a result of this effort.

We have selected and assimilated experiments done by numerous scientists and have used them to explain how cells work. In doing this, we have concentrated on animal cells because we know more about them. We have come to a deeper appreciation, while preparing this book, of the limitations in understanding the inner workings of the cell and have come to realize more than ever that we are, in these matters, still "looking through a glass darkly."

An explosively increasing body of knowledge about the cell and its organelles has become available through the diligent work of numerous biologists. Thus it is impractical to attempt to credit each of these scientists for all of their important contributions: The listed references are neither exhaustive nor are they necessarily the first report of a finding. Instead, references have been chosen to serve as reviews to which the interested student may turn. We apologize to all those slighted scientists whose names we have not cited and wish to make it clear that none of the important studies upon which this book is based was done by us, and hence all statements should be referenced. A truly complete bibliography would therefore yield a text referenced to the point of becoming unreadable by any student.

The authors wish to thank Mrs. Carlotta Roach for preparing all the photographs used in the text as well as for her many other services, the University of Washington Pathology Electron Microscope technicians for their technical assistance in preparing specimens for electron microscopy, Miss Virginia Wejak for typing the many stages of this manuscript, and Miss Leslie Caldwell and Joseph Ewing for taking many of the pictures used in Chapter I. We also wish to thank Miss Pat Phelps, Dr. C. Craig Tisher, Dr. Roger Bulger, Dr. Daniel Friend, Dr. Peter Satir, and Dr. Richard Sagebiel for reading the manuscript and providing helpful suggestions. Finally, we would like to thank Dr. Anita Hendrickson, Miss Mary Cahill, Mrs. Carlotta Roach, Dr. Douglas Kelly, Dr. Daniel Friend, Dr. James Koehler, Dr. Fred Silverblatt, Dr. T. L. Hayes, Dr. John Gilbert, Dr. Guido Tytgat, and Dr. Morris J. Karnovsky for allowing us to use their beautiful electron micrographs.

The reader will note that all diagrammatic figures appear near their references in the text but that all halftone figures (including, for example, all the electron micrographs) appear together following page 56.

The research of the authors has been supported in part by NIH grants AM–10922 and Career Development Award K04–AM–9878.

I

INTRODUCTION:
Tools for Examining
the Cytoplasm

The history of man's effort to describe the structure and understand the function of living material is a story of inventiveness, creativity, and technology. What biological scientists of every age have learned has been determined largely by the nature of the tools available to them. The development of the electron microscope and its application to the study of living material was therefore greeted with intense excitement by biologists. This powerful tool provides a bridge between the cells observed by the light microscopist and the molecules studied by the chemist. Using the electron microscope in conjunction with the techniques of the physiologist and the biochemist, scientists have begun to make meaningful correlations between the structure and the function of cells. The purpose of this book is to discuss some of the results of these studies as they apply to the functioning cytoplasm.

The results of these scientific explorations help to satisfy our curiosity about the world around us. In addition, we reap further benefit by applying this knowledge to the understanding and perhaps to the correction of alterations caused by injury and disease.

When only the light microscope was available for the study of cell structure, little was known about the substance of the cytoplasm. Biologists even disagreed about the existence of certain organelles such as the cell membrane and the Golgi apparatus because the details of these structures were below the limit of resolution of the light microscope (Table I–1). Later, when cells were viewed in the electron microscope, not only the organelles but also their intricate structural details were evident. Even single large molecules such as glycogen particles were resolved. Such data was of great importance to cell biologists who were interested in correlating cell structure with cell function. However, certain limitations are inherent in the use of the electron microscope for the study of cells. This is true first because the cells are subjected to several violent procedures. Usually they are cut from the animal, killed with a chemical fixative,

TABLE I-1

1 μ = 0.001 mm = 10,000 Å
1 μm = 10 Å
1 × 10⁻⁷ mm = 1 Å

Field of study	Anatomy	Histology	Cytology	Submicroscopic anatomy			Molecular level	Atom level
Basic unit	Organs	Tissues	Cells	Cell organelles			Small molecules	Atoms
	Tissues	Tissues	Bacteria	Viruses	Macromolecules			
Methods	Eye and simple lenses	Light microscopes	Ultraviolet phase	Electron microscopes			X-ray diffraction	
Electromagnetic spectrum	Radio waves	Infrared	v i s i b l e	Ultraviolet			X-rays	Gamma rays

Limit of eye — 0.1 mm
Limit of light microscope — 0.2 μm
Limit of electron microscope — 3 Å

1 mm	0.1 mm	0.01 mm	0.001 mm	0.0001 mm		0.001 μ	0.0001 μ
1,000 μ	100 μ	10 μ	1 μ	0.1 μ	0.01 μ		
10,000,000 Å	1,000,000 Å	100,000 Å	10,000 Å	1,000 Å	100 Å	10 Å	1 Å

and dehydrated. They are then embedded, sectioned, and viewed. Second, only a few cells are present in any given section; sampling a large amount of tissue becomes time-consuming. There are also limitations on interpreting the finest details observed in electron micrographs because the sections which are cut are thick with respect to the fine structural details being viewed.

Since the electron microscope has become such a vital research tool, it is of value to learn more about its design and operation.

COMPARISON OF LIGHT MICROSCOPES AND ELECTRON MICROSCOPES

Resolution. Viewing very small objects such as cells requires special instruments (see Table I–1). Before the advent of the electron microscope, the light microscope (Fig. I–1) was one of the most powerful tools available for examination of tissues and cells. However, the resolution of this instrument is limited and does not permit one to resolve the smaller components of the cell. The *limit of resolution* (an instrument's ability to form distinguishable images of objects separated by small distances) of the light microscope is expressed by Abbe's equation. This equation states that the limit of resolution equals a constant (0.612) times the wavelength of the light used, divided by the numerical aperture. The *numerical aperture* is a measure of the light-gathering power of the lens aperture and therefore equals the sin of the half-aperture angle times the refractive index of the medium between the specimen and the objective:

Abbe's Equation

$$\text{Resolution} = \frac{(0.612)\ (\text{wavelength of radiation used})}{(\text{index of refraction of medium between light and lens})\ (\sin\alpha\ \text{aperture angle of illuminating cone})}$$

$$\text{Resolution} = d = \frac{(0.612)\ (4,500)}{(1.4)\ (0.94)} \approx 2,000\ \mathring{A}\ \text{or}\ 0.2\ \mu$$

For the light microscope, the wavelength of visible light is approximately 4,500 Ångström units (violet light = 4,000 Ångström units, yellow-green light = 5,200 Ångström units), the aperture angle is close to 90°, and the numerical aperture of the best objective lenses is in the range of 1.3 to 1.4. The theoretical limit of resolution therefore equals approximately 2,000 Ångström units or 0.2 micron. (For a more rigorous derivation of this equation, see the excellent book by Wischnitzer.[37]) Since the numerator of Abbe's equation contains the wavelength of the radiation used, a decrease in this quantity (light of shorter wavelength) causes an increase in the resolution. Therefore, an ultraviolet microscope using a radiation of shorter wavelength (i.e., ultraviolet light = 2,500 Ångström units) would have increased resolving power. The limit of resolution of the ultraviolet microscope is approximately 1,000 Ångström units or 0.1 micron. In order to achieve a significant increase in resolving power, a shorter wavelength of radiation must be utilized. This was achieved with the development of the electron microscope.

Electrons under appropriate conditions display wave properties. The wavelength of an electron depends upon the accelerating potential which has been applied to it. When accelerated at 60 kilovolts (60,000 volts), the wavelength of an electron is 0.05 Ångström unit. This short wavelength should make electrons an ideal source of radiation for an instrument with high resolving power. The electron microscope (Fig. I–2) does employ electrons as a source of radiation and uses magnetic lenses to focus them. However, the entire theoretical increase in resolving power which should result from the much shorter wavelength of electrons is not realized in the electron microscope because the magnetic lenses which focus the electrons have certain inherent defects. Because these magnetic lenses are imperfect and often asymmetric, their numerical aperture is low. Whereas the numerical aperture of an objective lens for the light microscope is approximately 1.4, a magnetic lens has a numerical aperture of approximately 0.01 to 0.001. Despite this loss of potential resolving power due to magnetic lens defects, the limit of resolution of the electron microscope is markedly improved over that of the light microscope. A resolution of 3 to 5 Ångström units is claimed for the newest available electron microscopes. Although this resolution can be demonstrated with certain test substances, a resolution of approximately 15 Ångström units is obtained when sections of biological material are utilized.

Many similarities exist between light microscopes and electron microscopes. The components of an electron microscope are easier to understand when they are compared with those of a light microscope. Generally speaking, the elements of an electron microscope are inverted in their positions with respect to those of the light microscope.

Source of Radiation. The source of radiation for a light microscope is a light bulb located under the stage of the microscope or reflected from a distance by a substage mirror. The source of radiation for an electron microscope is an *electron gun* (cathode). The gun consists of a shielded tungsten filament located at the top of the instrument. The gun and its shield are connected to a high-voltage supply. When a current is passed through the pointed tungsten filament of the gun, heat is produced. As the filament becomes hotter, electrons in the metal gain sufficient energy to leave the filament and become free. The free electrons are attracted toward the anode, which is a grounded disc located a few centimeters beneath the tungsten cathode. Since the disc is at zero potential, it is positive with respect to the cathode gun, which is maintained between 40 and 100 kilovolts. This potential difference serves as the accelerating force for the electrons.

Condenser Lens. The condenser lens of the light microscope is positioned above the light source. It consists of a combination of glass lenses which regulate the intensity of the light and focus it on the specimen. The condenser lens of the electron microscope is an electromagnetic lens situated beneath the anode. It functions in a similar manner by regulating the intensity of the electron beam and focusing it upon the specimen.

Specimen. For light microscopy, the tissue section is placed on a supporting glass slide, which is inserted on top of the microscope stage above the condenser lens. These tissue sections are generally between 1 and 7 microns in thickness. For electron microscopy the specimen is inserted into a chamber in the column of the instrument beneath the condenser lens. It is therefore situated close to the focal plane of the objective lens. Sections for the electron microscope consist of a very thin (approximately 200 to 1,000 Ångström units thick) plastic-embedded tissue. These are placed upon copper mesh grids for support. The areas of the sections lying over the holes of the copper grid are viewed.

Contrast. Since biological specimens are largely transparent in visible light, contrast differences must be produced for viewing with a light microscope. Two ways of achieving sufficient contrast are routinely utilized: introduction of *stains* into tissue and introduction of *phase changes* in the light passing through the tissue. Staining of the tissue with colored dye is done to increase contrast in the material to be viewed in a conventional light microscope. The dyes, preferentially bound to certain tissue components, absorb light of specific wavelengths. Unstained material does not absorb light differentially, but the material can affect the light passing through it by retarding some "wave trains" more than others, therefore changing the phase of the light waves. Although these phase differences are not perceptible to the eye, a *phase microscope* can convert these phase differences into differences in contrast. This type of microscope is particularly useful for viewing living material.

The production of contrast in the electron microscope involves a different process than that used in the light microscope. Electrons emitted from the filament are attracted to the anode disc. Those electrons which pass through the hole in the disc glide down the column of the electron microscope until they reach the level of the specimen. In the specimen the electrons interact with the tissue and *scattering* occurs. When the electrons interact or collide with the heavy nucleus of an atom, *elastic scattering* takes place. The electrons change in direction without appreciable loss of energy because little energy is transferred to the very large nucleus. The change in direction which occurs when electrons interact with a heavy nucleus causes a deletion of electrons in that area of the image. Therefore, such scattering contributes to the formation of the image on the screen or on the film. In the second kind of scattering, called *inelastic scattering,* beam electrons interact with the orbiting electrons of atoms in the specimen. During this type of scattering there is a decrease in the energy of the electrons and frequently a change in their direction. Because electrons with decreased energies sometimes contribute to the formation of an image, inelastic scattering gives rise to peripheral blurring. Therefore, a specimen's ability to scatter electrons is related to the mass density of the material within it. For this reason, solutions of heavy metal compounds are used as stains to increase the mass in local regions of the specimen and thereby enhance contrast.

Objective Lens. In the light microscope, the objective lens is located above the specimen. It consists of a series of glass lenses which produce the magnified initial image. Several objectives ranging in magnifying power can be rotated into position. The most commonly used lenses magnify the tissue preparation 10, 40, or 100 times. The objective lens of the electron microscope also produces the initial magnified image. However, this lens is electromagnetic and lies directly beneath the specimen grid. The objective lens in both kinds of microscopes produces the most critical image of the specimen. Since additional magnification of this image cannot improve the resolution, it is important that the objective lens be as free of imperfections as possible.

In the electron microscope an intense magnetic field must be produced within the objective lens in order to produce a highly magnified image. To accomplish this, two soft iron pole pieces are placed inside the objective lens. Pole pieces may, however, have imperfections within them and their metal content may not be homogeneous. These imperfections, as well as the presence of certain contaminating materials within the column of the electron microscope, can lead to the production of an asymmetrical magnetic field in the objective lens, which results in a poor initial image (*astigmatism*). It is possible to correct for this astigmatism by superimposing a counteracting magnetic field upon the objective lens which opposes the existing asymmetry in the lens. This is done by positioning within the lens a device called a stigmator, which allows one to compensate for the asymmetry.

Projector. The next functional component of the light microscope is the ocular or eyepiece lens. It consists of a series of glass lenses arranged to magnify a portion of the image produced by the objective lens and thus forms the final image. The projector lens of an electron microscope is an electromagnetic lens, which serves the same function by magnifying the image produced by the objective lens.

Final Image. In a light microscope the final image that is produced can be projected directly onto the retina of the eye, or it can be projected onto a photographic plate or film and thus be permanently recorded. In an electron microscope, the final image cannot be projected directly onto the eye because the image is formed by the presence or absence of electrons to which the eye is not sensitive. The image is therefore projected onto a fluorescent screen. When the electrons from the beam strike the phosphor of the screen, photons are emitted and produce a positive visible image of the specimen. The electrons may also be allowed to bombard a photographic film or plate. In this case they produce a latent image, which can be developed to give a negative image of the specimen. This negative can be enlarged and printed in a typical photographic manner (Fig. I–3).

ELECTRON MICROSCOPE COLUMN

The column of an electron microscope (Fig. I–2), through which the electrons move, is maintained under vacuum. Operation of the electron microscope under vacuum is essential because an electron beam can be produced only in a vacuum. In air, electrons travel only short distances because they are stopped by collisions with gas molecules. When most of the gas molecules have been pumped out of the column, fewer collisions occur. A good vacuum also increases the lifetime of the filament; when air is present within the column, tungsten oxides form eroding the filament. The vacuum also decreases the tendency for a discharge to occur between the cathode and the anode. The vacuum is produced and maintained by two types of pumps located in the electron microscope. The *forepump*, which is a mechanical pump, easily moves large volumes of air from the column and can produce the vacuum of 10^{-2} mm of mercury. This vacuum is not sufficient for adequate operation of the electron microscope, so a second pump, an *oil diffusion pump*, has been incorporated into the system. It operates sequentially with the mechanical forepump and produces and maintains the vacuum at 10^{-4} mm of mercury or better during operation of the electron microscope.

SPECIMEN PREPARATION FOR THE ELECTRON MICROSCOPE

Tissue specimens prepared for electron microscopy should conform to the following requirements: (1) they must be fixed in a manner that maintains a state as nearly identical to that found in living material as is possible; (2) they must be altered as little as possible during subsequent preparation; (3) the sections must be embedded in material that is able to withstand the effects of a vacuum and an electron beam; (4) they must be sectioned thin enough to allow penetration of the electron beam.

Fixation. In order to preserve the structure of cells and tissues as closely as possible to that found in the living state, a variety of chemical fixatives has been employed.[4] Except for osmium tetroxide, the fixatives traditionally used for light microscopy at first appeared to be generally unsuccessful when used in electron microscopy. Osmium tetroxide gained wide acceptance and was utilized almost exclusively for most of the early, descriptive, electron microscopical studies of cells. However, later investigations employed other fixative solutions that appeared satisfactory. These included potassium permanganate,[18] formaldehyde,[12] and other aldehydes such as glutaraldehyde.[17,28] Chemical fixatives appear to stabilize structures by the formation of cross-links between compounds in the specimen. The compounds that are cross-linked are generally proteins and lipids. The use of a variety of fixatives on a given tissue has frequently revealed differences in structure that appear to be related to the fixative used. For example, in the ciliary epithelium of the eye, chains of vesicles have been seen in the basal cytoplasm of the cells after fixation in solutions containing osmium tetroxide, whereas sheets of membrane-bounded interdigitating processes were seen after fixation with glutaraldehyde.[34] Such results emphasize the fact that the alterations which occur in living tissues during fixation are not well known and can profoundly affect various cell structures. Therefore, interpretations of electron micrographs must be approached with caution. Material fixed in aldehydes is generally postfixed in osmium tetroxide-containing solutions before dehydration and embedding because the osmium tetroxide acts as a tissue stain. Aldehyde fixatives offer an advantage in that they do not inactivate all the enzymes in a tissue. Therefore, it is possible to apply histochemical reactions and localize certain cellular enzymes in aldehyde-fixed material. Modifying some of these histochemical techniques for use in electron microscopy makes it possible to visualize specific subcellular sites where a particular enzyme is located.

The method of fixative application is also important and greatly affects the morphology of the tissue. Usually, tissue is excised from the animal and cut into small pieces before being placed into the fixative solution. This procedure may cause changes in tissue morphology. If one is preparing to fix brain tissue which is contained within the skull, many cellular changes can occur during the lengthy process of obtaining the tissue.[25] The same is true for organs which depend upon the blood supply for maintenance of their normal morphology, as appears to be the case with the mammalian kidney. When diced blocks of kidney tissue are fixed by immersion, the lumens of most of the tubules are closed, whereas in the living state the lumens are open. To avoid the difficulties inherent in fixing excised tissue, fixative solutions can be dripped onto the surface of organs or flooded over thin tissue layers. In these cases, only a thin layer of tissue is adequately fixed for study. This process works well only for thin sheets of tissue or for studies of the surface cells of organs. However, if one is interested in fixing entire organs, perfusing the fixative solutions through the blood vessels of the animal appears to be the best technique. Such a procedure has been used in preserving tissue from the central nervous system[25] and from the kidney.[10,20]

All the methods described so far involve the interaction of the tissue with a chemical solution. Alternative methods of preserving tissue have been devised by a number of workers and have great applicability. Tissue which has been rapidly frozen and dried while maintained in the cold may be viewed in the electron microscope.[2,31] These pieces of tissue have not been in contact with any chemical fixatives. Alternatively, the details present in the frozen tissue can be viewed by utilizing a method called freeze-etching. The tissue is rapidly frozen and then fractured to form a new surface. The ice in the specimen can be allowed to sublimate, creating an etching effect in areas of high water content in the cells, thus revealing surfaces of cell membranes. A metal layer is evaporated over the specimen in a vacuum to produce a replica of this surface structure. This replica produces contrast when viewed in the scope. A backing of carbon is also evaporated on the replica for reinforcement. The tissue is then removed from the replica and the latter is viewed in the electron microscope.[22,23] It is also possible to dehydrate unfixed tissues using inert solvents such as ethylene glycol or glycerol instead of water.[26] The inert substance is added in gradually increasing concentrations, and it eventually displaces all the water molecules in the tissue, thereby immobilizing the tissue macromolecules. These techniques of preparing tissue without chemical fixation provide alternative methods of evaluating tissue structure. A comparison of tissue prepared by these methods with tissue fixed chemically can lead to an increased knowledge of cellular structure in the living animal. Figures I–4 through I–7 compare the image of a nucleated red blood cell produced by conventional chemical fixation (Fig. I–4), by freeze-etching (Fig. I–5), by air drying and shadowing (Fig. I–6), and by negative staining (Fig. I–7).

Embedding. After completion of chemical fixation, water in the specimen is replaced by a material which is miscible with the embedding medium. For routine electron microscopy, the tissue is placed in solutions containing increasing concentrations of alcohol. In this dehydration procedure the alcohol replaces the water molecules in the tissue (Fig. I–8). After the water has been removed, the tissue is placed into a liquid plastic embedding medium (Fig. I–9). The embedding medium infiltrates the tissue, and when this process is completed the infiltrated tissue is hardened. An epoxy resin is the most commonly used embedding medium for electron microscopy. The liquid epoxy containing the tissue specimen is polymerized by heat and a solid transparent plastic block results.[19] The solid plastic supports the tissue so that it will withstand the subsequent cutting and bombardment by electrons from the electron beam.

Sectioning and Staining. The plastic-embedded capsule containing the tissue is trimmed to a small size with a razor blade (Fig. I–10). It is then mounted in a microtome and thin sections are cut (Fig. I–11). For use in electron microscopy, ultramicrotomes have been specifically designed. The sections are cut using glass or diamond knives. Glass knives are made just before using by scoring and breaking pieces of glass; sharpened diamond knives are commercially available. As the thin sections are cut they are floated off the knife edge onto the surface of the water contained in a trough affixed to the knife. The approximate thickness of the thin sections can be estimated visually by interference colors reflected from their surfaces. Sections that are between 100 and 1,000 Ångström units are useful in ordinary electron microscopy. The floating ribbons of sections are then picked up on small, round, copper mesh grids. Once on the grids, the sections may be viewed as they are or they may be treated with heavy metal staining solutions. Uranyl acetate[35] and/or lead salts [21,35] are commonly used to stain these thin sections. Thicker sections (1 μ) can be cut and placed on glass slides for viewing in the light microscope (Fig. I–12).

Negative Staining of Molecules, Viruses, and Isolated Cell Organelles. In positive staining procedures, the sections are treated with solutions containing heavy metals. These solutions tend to increase the mass density of specific tissue structures and thereby increase the contrast of the tissue. Another technique, called *negative staining,* produces increased contrast by the formation of an electron-opaque layer around the structure to be studied. This technique has been particularly useful in studying viruses and molecules. Although the electron stain can fill cavities and indentations, it does not penetrate hydrophobic regions of the structure and these therefore appear electron lucent. Because the contrast between the negative stain and the substance is great, the resolution of this technique exceeds that found in tissue sections. In practice, the substance to be studied is mixed with a solution containing the negative stain and sprayed on grids for viewing. The negative stains most commonly used are potassium phosphotungstate and uranyl acetate.

TECHNIQUES USED IN CONJUNCTION WITH THE ELECTRON MICROSCOPE

The commerical production of electron microscopes and the technical improvements which allowed sections of biological materials to be viewed in them allowed use of the instrument to describe the normal structure of many animal cells. Observations have been made of structural changes seen in diseased tissue. Investigations have also been conducted on tissue which had been experimentally altered in some manner, either by a change in its physiological state or by injury. Although these morphological findings have added greatly to our knowledge, the use of the electron microscope in conjunction with other biological techniques has contributed even more to our understanding of how the cell functions.

Localization of Substances at a Subcellular Level. *Cytochemistry.* The identification and localization of substances such as enzymes within cells or tissues are subject to many technical problems. Before the electron microscope can be used for the detection of specific subcellular sites, strict requirements must be met. The requirements necessary for success are (1) the fixation must be adequate so that one can resolve the structures present; (2) the fixative must prevent the diffusion of the substance that is to be localized; (3) the fixative must not destroy the chemical reactivity of the substance to be localized; (4) the fixative should also block nonspecific absorption of the particular substance to be measured or the marking agent onto some other structure; (5) the reaction between the substance to be localized and the marking agent must be specific; and (6) the reaction product must be insoluble and electron dense in order to be seen in the electron microscope.

Nucleic acids[1,13,32,36] were some of the first compounds localized by electron microscopical cytochemistry. The localization of additional substances at the ultrastructural level generally resulted from the modification of existing light microscopical techniques, making them applicable to electron microscopy. It has therefore been possible, using these modified techniques, to identify certain enzymes, mucosubstances, aldehydes, and antibodies in cells.

The localization of certain specific enzymes became more feasible with the use of aldehyde fixatives.[12,28] These fixatives do not cause total inactivation of all enzymes. Some enzymes remain active in fixed tissue. A few enzymes will react with the appropriate substrate to produce a particular product which in certain cases can be made electron opaque, often by its reaction with a metal salt such as lead phosphate, which is used in the Gomori method for acid phosphatase.[6] In some cases, an insoluble nonmetallic compound of high molecular weight is used, as in the azo dye method.[29]

Immunochemistry. Immunochemistry is another important technique employed for the localization of large molecules. Antibodies are prepared against a specific tissue antigen. These antibodies are then coupled to a large tracer molecule, which can be visualized in thin tissue sections prepared for electron microscopy.[30] Ferritin is frequently used to label antibodies because it can be identified by its characteristic structure. More recently, however, antibodies also have been labeled with a smaller enzyme, horseradish peroxidase.[24] This smaller marker has the advantage of being less likely to affect the normal action of the antibody molecule (i.e., in combining with its specific tissue antigen). Because horseradish peroxidase is an enzyme, it can be localized in tissue following its reaction with a proper substrate (in this case, H_2O_2, and an electron donor, diaminobenzidine). The product of this reaction is made electron opaque by postfixation in osmium tetroxide. Important information about the function of cells is being derived as these procedures are being further refined and applied in the study of a wide variety of tissue.

Tracers. In order to study how large molecules are handled in the living animal, a variety of tracer particles have been used experimentally. These include such compounds as ferritin, colloidal gold, and Thorotrast. A number of smaller particles (i.e., enzymes with peroxidase activity)[7,8,9,33] has now also become available. These smaller tracers can be identified in minute quantities in tissue because of the enzymatic activity of the peroxidases. Such enzymatic proteins permit the study of mechanisms whereby cells handle proteins of various sizes (Fig. I–13).

Horseradish peroxidase is a small tracer particle presently being used and has a molecular weight of approximately 40,000.[15] Lactoperoxidase, with a molecular weight of 82,000, is similar in size to albumin and can be visualized in a similar manner in electron micrographs.[9,27] Human myeloperoxidase has a molecular weight of 160,000 and may be used as a tracer of large proteins. These compounds have already provided much information on capillary permeability,[14] protein filtration in the kidney,[8] and protein uptake by cells.[7] The continued use of these tracers should provide more information on protein metabolism and transport by various cells and tissues.

Localization of Ions by Precipitation Techniques. Techniques to localize the position of various ions in tissue would be valuable in understanding cell function. Attempts have been made to precipitate sodium and chloride ions in their normal position in tissue and to view the precipitate using an electron microscope.[16] Although careful control experiments demonstrating the reliability of these techniques have not been done, the significance of these techniques may be great.

Radioautography. Radioautography is another technique which may be used in conjunction with electron microscopy. The basic principle used in this procedure involves the incorporation of a radioactive isotope of an element into a particular chemical substance within the cell. Since the radioactive isotope has a different (and less stable) atomic structure than the element itself, it acts as a marker by emitting radiation which can be detected. Sections of tissue containing the isotope are coated with a thin layer of photographic emulsion. These coated sections are then stored in the dark for a length of time. During this period, ionizing radiation is emitted as the radioactive isotope decays. As the emitted radiation collides with silver halide ions in the overlying photographic emulsion, a latent image is formed over the specific area where the marked chemical substance is located within the cell. After a sufficient exposure period, the latent image is developed by photographic processing. The resulting image consists of metallic silver, formed by the reduction of the silver halide at the site of the emitted radiation. This procedure was used very successfully in conjunction with electron microscopy by Caro[3] in 1961 to follow the synthesis of protein by pancreatic acinar cells.

Cell Fractionation Procedures. Electron microscopy has also been used in conjunction with cell fractionation procedures. Such studies have yielded important information about the function of various cellular components because it is possible to use the electron microscope appearance of a fraction as a criterion of its purity. In this way, one can test whether one known cell constituent is associated with a known biochemical reaction.

The most common fractionation procedure begins with the homogenation (or grinding) of tissue in a homogenizer. The disrupted material is then treated in one of two ways. One method is known as *differential ultracentrifugation*. In this procedure the homogenized material is placed on the top of a sucrose solution in a test tube and centrifuged at a series of increasing speeds.[5,11] After each centrifugation, the pellet of material in the bottom of the test tube is recovered. These pellets may then be used for correlated biochemical and morphological studies.

The second method used in studying the homogenized cell material is known as *density gradient centrifugation*. In this case the homogenate is put into a tube on top of a stabilized gradient consisting of increasing concentrations of a substance such as sucrose and the tube is then centrifuged. Particles from the homogenate descend in the gradient and come to rest where the density of the gradient in the tube is equal to their own density. The variation in density of different cell components causes a layering or stratification of the components. Layers from the gradient can be analyzed separately and studied by biochemical as well as morphological procedures.

SCANNING ELECTRON MICROSCOPES

In conventional transmission electron microscopy (described earlier) very thin sections must be utilized because the image is formed by electrons which pass through the specimen. A new type of instrument, called the scanning microscope, has been devised for the direct examination of the surfaces of specimens (Figs. I–14 and I–15). As the specimen is scanned by an electron beam, secondary electron emission occurs from the specimen itself. These liberated electrons are utilized to reproduce the topography, or surface detail, of the specimen. The scanning microscope has a depth of focus hundreds of times greater than even a conventional light microscope.

HIGH-VOLTAGE ELECTRON MICROSCOPES

One factor which limits resolution of conventional electron microscopes is chromatic aberration. This aberration can be decreased if the accelerating voltage of the electrons is increased. In high-voltage electron microscopes, the accelerating voltages are in the range of 1 million electron volts instead of 50,000 to 100,000 electron volts. The resolution obtained with these new high-voltage instruments should be better than that obtained with conventional electron microscopes. The increased energy of the electrons (and therefore the increased penetration power) should allow the use of thicker sections of tissue. The use of thicker sections allows one to avoid painstaking serial reconstruction of the thinner sections for the understanding of complex tissue morphology. Whole living organisms may someday be viewed within a chamber in a high-voltage microscope. It is also conceivable that the use of this instrument might result in a decrease in damage from the electron beam. However, high-voltage electron microscopes have not yet been utilized to any great degree by biologists.

As more instruments become available for use in solving biological problems, their apparent potential may be fulfilled.

REFERENCES

[1] Peter Albersheim and Ursula Killias,"The Use of Bismuth as an Electron Stain for Nucleic Acids," *J. Cell Biol.*, 17 (1963), 93–103.

[2] R. R. Bensley and N. L. Hoerr, "Studies on Cell Structure by the Freezing-Drying Method. V. The Chemical Basis of the Organization of the Cell," *Anat. Rec.*, 60 (1934), 251–266.

[3] L. G. Caro, "Electron Microscopic Radioautography of Thin Sections: The Golgi Zone as a Site of Protein Concentration in Pancreatic Acinar Cells," *J. Biophys. Biochem. Cytol.*, 10 (1961), 37–46.

[4] A. Claude and E. F. Fullam, "The Preparation of Sections of Guinea Pig Liver for Electron Microscopy," *J. Exp. Med.*, 83 (1946), 499–504.

[5] Albert Claude, "Fractionation of Mammalian Liver Cells by Differential Centrifugation. I. Problems, Methods and Preparation of Extract," *J. Exp. Med.*, 84 (1946), 51–59.

[6] George Gomori, *Microscopic Histochemistry; Principles and Practice* (Chicago: University of Chicago Press, 1952).

[7] R. C. Graham and M. J. Karnovsky, "The Early Stages of Absorption of Injected Horseradish Peroxidase in the Proximal Tubules of Mouse Kidney: Ultrastructural Cytochemistry by a New Technique," *J. Histochem. Cytochem.*, 14 (1966), 291–302.

[8] R. C. Graham and M. J. Karnovsky, "Glomerular Permeability. Ultrastructural Cytochemical Studies Using Peroxidases as Protein Tracers," *J. Exp. Med.*, 124 (1966), 1123–1134.

[9] R. C. Graham and R. W. Kellermeyer, "Bovine Lactoperoxidase as a Cytochemical Protein Tracer for Electron Microscopy," *J. Histochem. Cytochem.*, 16 (1968), 275–278.

[10] L. D. Griffith, R. E. Bulger, and B. F. Trump, "The Ultrastructure of the Functioning Kidney," *Lab. Invest.*, 16 (1967), 220–246.

[11]G. H. Hogeboom, W. C. Schneider, and George E. Palade, "Cytochemical Studies of Mammalian Tissues. I. Isolation of Intact Mitochondria from Rat Liver; Some Biochemical Properties of Mitochondria and Submicroscopic Particulate Material," *J. Biol. Chem.*, 172 (1948), 619–635.

[12]S. J. Holt and R. M. Hicks, "Studies on Formalin Fixation for Electron Microscopy and Cytochemical Staining Purposes," *J. Biophys. Biochem. Cytol.*, 11 (1961), 31–45.

[13]H. E. Huxley and G. Zubay, "Preferential Staining of Nucleic Acid-Containing Structures for Electron Microscopy," *J. Biophys. Biochem. Cytol.*, 11 (1961), 273–296.

[14]M. J. Karnovsky, "The Ultrastructural Basis of Transcapillary Exchanges," *J. Gen. Physiol.*, 52 (1968), 64s–95s.

[15]D. Keilin and E. F. Hartree, "Purification of Horseradish Peroxidase and Comparison of Its Properties with Those of Catalase and Methaemoglobin," *Biochem. J.*, 49 (1951), 88–104.

[16]H. Komnick, "Elektronen Mikroskopische Lokalisation von Na^+ und Cl^- in Zellen und Geweben," *Protoplasma*, 55 (1962), 414.

[17]J. H. Luft, "The Use of Acrolein as a Fixative for Light and Electron Microscopy," *Anat. Rec.*, 133 (1959), 3055.

[18]J. H. Luft, "Permanganate—A New Fixative for Electron Microscopy," *J. Biophys. Biochem. Cytol.*, 2 (1956), 799–801.

[19]J. H. Luft, "Improvements in Epoxy Resin Embedding Methods," *J. Biophys. Biochem. Cytol.*, 9 (1961), 409–414.

[20]A. B. Maunsbach, "The Influence of Different Fixatives and Fixation Methods on the Ultrastructure of Rat Kidney Proximal Tubule Cells. I. Comparison of Different Perfusion Fixation Methods and of Glutaraldehyde, Formaldehyde and Osmium Tetroxide Fixatives," *J. Ultrastruct. Res.*, 15 (1966), 242–282.

[21]Giuseppe Millonig, "A Modified Procedure for Lead Staining of Thin Sections," *J. Biophys. Biochem. Cytol.*, 11(1961), 736–739.

[22]H. Moor and K. Mühlethaler, "Fine Structure in Frozen-Etched Yeast Cells," *J. Cell Biol.*, 17 (1963), 609–628.

[23]H. Moor, K. Mühlethaler, H. Waldner, and A. Frey-Wyssling, "A New Freezing-Ultramicrotome," *J. Biophys. Biochem. Cytol.*, 10 (1961), 1–14.

[24]P. K. Nakane and G. B. Pierce, Jr., "Enzyme-Labeled Antibodies: Preparation and Application for the Localization of Antigens," *J. Histochem. Cytochem.*, 14 (1966), 929–931.

[25]S. L. Palay, S. M. McGee-Russell, Spencer Gordon, Jr., and M. A. Grillo, "Fixation of Neural Tissues for Electron Microscopy by Perfusion with Solutions of Osmium Tetroxide," *J. Cell Biol.*, 12 (1962), 385–410.

[26]D. C. Pease, "The Preservation of Unfixed Cytological Detail by Dehydration with 'Inert' Agents," *J. Ultrastruct. Res.*, 14 (1966), 356–378.

[27]B. D. Polis and H. W. Shmukler, "Crystalline Lactoperoxidase. I. Isolation by Displacement Chromatography. II. Physicochemical and Enzymatic Properties," *J. Biol. Chem.*, 201 (1953), 475–500.

[28]D. D. Sabatini, Klaus Bensch, and R.J. Barrnett, "Cytochemistry and Electron Microscopy. The Preservation of Cellular Ultrastructure and Enzymatic Activity by Aldehyde Fixation," *J. Cell Biol.*, 17 (1963), 19–58.

[29]A. W. Sedar and C. G. Rosa, "Cytochemical Demonstration of the Succinic Dehydrogenase System with the Electron Microscope Using Nitro-Blue Tetrazolium," *J. Ultrastruct. Res.*, 5 (1961), 226–243.

[30]S. J. Singer, "Preparation of an Electron-Dense Antibody Conjugate," *Nature* (London), 183 (1959), 1523–1524.

[31]F. S. Sjöstrand and R. F. Baker, "Fixation by Freezing-Drying for Electron Microscopy of Tissue Cells," *J. Ultrastruct. Res.*, 1 (1958), 239–246.

[32]Walther Stoeckenius, "Electron Microscopy of DNA Molecules 'Stained' with Heavy Metal Salts," *J. Biophys. Biochem. Cytol.*, 11 (1961), 297–310.

[33]W. Straus, "Rapid Cytochemical Identification of Phagosomes in Various Tissues of the Rat and Their Differentiation from Mitochondria by the Peroxidase Method," *J. Biophys. Biochem. Cytol.*, 5 (1959), 193–204.

[34]J. M. Tormey, "Differences in Membrane Configuration between Osmium Tetroxide-Fixed and Glutaraldehyde-Fixed Ciliary Epithelium" *J. Cell Biol.*, 23 (1964), 658–664.

[35]M. L. Watson, "Staining of Tissue Sections for Electron Microscopy with Heavy Metals," *J. Biophys. Biochem. Cytol.*, 4 (1958), 475–478.

[36]M. L. Watson and W. G. Aldridge, "Methods for the Use of Indium as an Electron Stain for Nucleic Acids," *J. Biophys. Biochem. Cytol.*, 11 (1961), 257–272.

[37]Saul Wischnitzer, *Introduction to Electron Microscopy* (New York: Pergamon Press, Inc., 1962).

II

ENERGY PRODUCTION AND USE

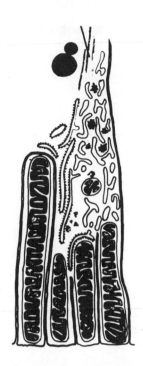

ENERGY AND METABOLISM

Energy sustains the living world. In cells energy is stored as potential energy in chemical compounds. When these chemical compounds are broken down, the energy is released to do work and to perform syntheses. Ultimately it ends up in products of low energy content, or is dissipated as heat. Cells require a constant supply of energy in order to maintain their life processes. They have the ability to trap energy, store it, and then, when the occasion demands, transform it into kinetic energy through biochemical reactions.

Metabolism, the sum of all chemical reactions carried out by cells, includes catabolic processes which break down foodstuffs and anabolic processes which synthesize new compounds. The former result in a liberation of energy (*exergonic reactions*), while the latter consume energy (*endergonic reactions*). In plants, the most important anabolic process, *photosynthesis,* involves trapping of the sun's energy by chlorophyll. A complex series of reactions is initiated whereby radiant energy is transformed and stored as carbohydrate. The following equation summarizes the general reaction of photosynthesis:

$$CO_2 + 2H_2O \xrightarrow{\quad h\nu \quad} CH_2O + H_2O + O_2$$

photon of light

Carbohydrates stored in plants include starch and sucrose. These compounds, important foods for animals, are broken down, and energy is released that is used to carry out life functions. In this chapter we review briefly how cells are able to unlock and use chemical energy. We reserve part of our discussion of how cells synthesize complex macromolecules for later chapters. However, it is important to realize that the pathways mentioned in this chapter are, for the most part, readily reversible, and that they can be used for synthesis if energy is supplied to the cell.

ENZYMES

A remarkable feature of cells is their ability to carry out metabolic processes at low temperatures. These chemical reactions occur within a narrow range of acidity (expressed as pH), and in a medium having a low ionic strength, in contrast to most laboratory reaction, where high temperatures and more extreme conditions are required to drive chemical reactions to completion. This characteristic property of living cells is made possible by proteins acting as enzymes.[2] All enzymes are protein, but it is not clear whether all structural proteins also possess enzymatic activity. In recent years, studies employing the electron microscope and other analytical tools have tended to obscure any critical differences between structural and biochemical features of cellular macromolecules such as enzymes. Specific enzymes comprise portions of the external cell membrane and others are part of the membranes of organelles such as the endoplasmic reticulum and mitochondria. Enzymes are also present in the cytoplasm of cells, within the matrix of mitochondria, and within other cellular components such as lysosomes and peroxisomes.

Enzymes act as catalysts by speeding up the rate of biochemical reactions. They do this by lowering the level of energy normally required to bring a reactive substance into an *activated state*. Only after activation can the reaction proceed with a loss of free energy. The change in free energy, ΔF, is a measure of the difference between the energy levels of the reactant and the product. Figure II–1 illustrates the activated state. A reaction proceeds spontaneously only if it is accompanied by a loss of free energy. ΔF is then negative (an exergonic reaction). In an endergonic reaction (going from B to A in Fig. II–1) free energy must be put into the system before the reaction can take place and ΔF is positive. If ΔF is zero, the system is at equilibrium.

All proteins and therefore all enzymes have a particular *primary structure*, that is, they are composed of a genetically determined specific sequence of amino acids. In addition, proteins have *secondary* and *tertiary structures* resulting from intramolecular interactions that give three dimensional configuration to the amino acid string. Finally, some proteins contain more than one polypeptide chain. The association of two or more

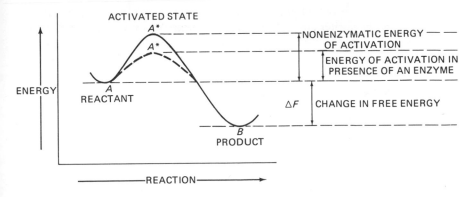

FIGURE II–1. A comparison of the energy of activation for enzymatic and nonenzymatic chemical reactions.

polypeptide chains to form such a protein molecule is called *quaternary structure*. Many enzymes displaying quaternary structure are able to regulate and control reactions by undergoing structural changes when they interact with substrates. (The importance of protein structure becomes even more evident when we discuss metabolic regulation later in this chapter.) These structural characteristics are important in determining the catalytic properties of an enzyme molecule and are sometimes modifiable within cells.

The surfaces of enzymes have *active sites* where *substrates*, upon which enzymes act, are bound. The active sites, formed by a folding of the large enzyme molecule, vary in their specificity. In order to react with an enzyme, the substrate must fit the active site in a complementary way, much as a key fits a lock. Some enzymes show absolute specificity and bind only one substrate, while others act upon a variety of similar chemical compounds. During the binding process, the bonds of the substrate molecule are strained so that transformation into the product can occur. When the substrate has been released the enzyme can return to its original configuration and the active site is ready to interact with a second substrate molecule. Each enzyme has a pH at which its activity is optimal; some enzymes work in a slightly acid range, while others require weakly alkaline conditions. Most mammalian enzymes show maximal activity at 37°C (mammalian body temperature). As temperature increases, the rate of reaction also increases, doubling for each 10-degree rise to the point where denaturation begins. Extremes in pH and ionic strength also destroy these proteins. However, some enzymes can refold spontaneously and regain activity when the denaturing agent is removed.

Inactive forms of enzymes, called *zymogens*, exist in some cells. They must be activated before they can catalyze reactions. This is usually accomplished by other enzymes, or by changes in pH, which split off a portion of the molecule. The cleavage unmasks or creates the active sites of the enzyme, rendering it active.

ENZYME–SUBSTRATE REACTIONS

The activity of an enzyme is a measure of its ability to transform a substrate into various products (P) (Fig. II–2). It is characteristic of enzyme-catalyzed reactions that the substrate first becomes bound to the surface of the enzyme to form an activated *enzyme–substrate complex* (ES*). This binding may be transitory but it is specific and occurs at the active site of the enzyme. Since the enzyme (E) must bind the substrate (S), the reaction rate depends upon the relative concentrations of enzyme and substrate.

Graphing the velocity of enzyme–substrate reactions under experimental laboratory conditions demonstrates some interesting kinetic relationships (Fig. II–3). High concentration of enzyme relative to substrate results in high reaction velocity. This is true, since there are many enzyme molecules with available active sites waiting to bind the substrate. Therefore, the high initial velocity plots as a steep slope. The pitch of the slope is a rough indication of the affinity of the enzyme for the substrate; the steeper the slope, the greater the affinity. The addition of more substrate eventually results in a saturation of all enzyme active sites and a maximum velocity (Vmax) is reached. A plateau then occurs, and increasing the substrate concentration further cannot affect the reaction. At this limiting velocity, the activity of the enzyme is proportional to its concentration.

Enzymes often are named by adding the suffix *ase* to the substrate upon which they act. For example, the enzyme involved in breaking the bond of the adenosine triphosphate (ATP) molecule is called ATPase.

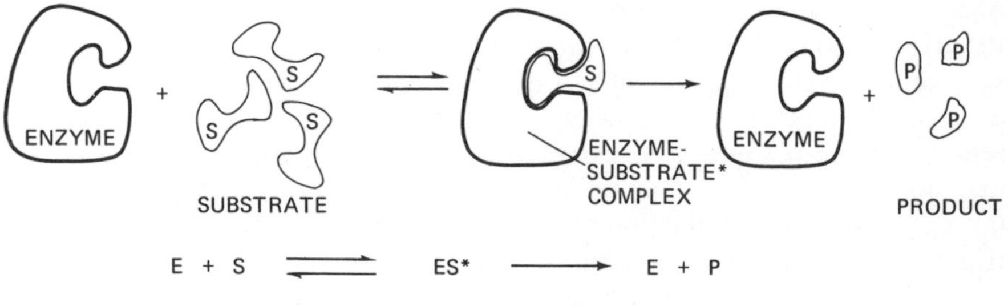

$$E + S \rightleftharpoons ES^* \longrightarrow E + P$$

FIGURE II–2. Enzyme–substrate interaction. In enzyme-catalyzed reactions the substrate first becomes bound to the surface of the enzyme to form an activated enzyme–substrate complex which subsequently dissociates to form enzyme and a product.

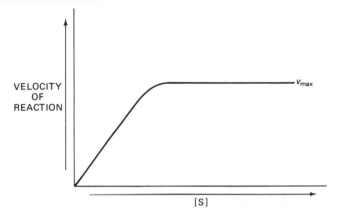

FIGURE II–3. This graph shows the relationship between substrate concentration $\lfloor S \rfloor$ and the initial velocity of reaction.

COUPLED REACTIONS

In the course of an enzyme reaction the substrate is converted into one or more products, which may in turn serve as substrates for other enzymatic reactions. As a result, biochemical reactions become "coupled" to one another. In living systems, it is common to find energy-supplying (exergonic) reactions coupled with energy-utilizing (endergonic) reactions. The mechanism of energy coupling requires a chemical compound common to both reactions.

ADENOSINE TRIPHOSPHATE (ATP) AND HIGH-ENERGY DONORS

In cells, the most important energy-carrying compound is adenosine triphosphate (ATP). The main pathways for energy storage or utilization in cells—photosynthesis, glycolysis, and oxidative phosphorylation—all generate ATP with varying efficiency. ATP consists of the purine base adenine, the five-carbon sugar ribose, and three phosphoric acid residues bonded to one another (Fig. II–4). ATP is able to transfer one or sometimes two of its end phosphate groups to another compound. In these transphosphorylation reactions the acceptor compounds have energy states similar to that of ATP, so a high-energy bond still exists. The subsequent release of this phosphate group from the second compound supplies the energy necessary for coupling of certain biochemical reactions. The triphosphates of uridine (UTP), cytidine (CTP), and guanosine (GTP) are other important high-energy donors. They function in the synthesis of important products such as glycogen, phospholipids, carbohydrates, and proteins. Phosphocreatine, phosphoenolpyruvic acid, and acetyl phosphate also have high-energy bonds that serve to supply energy for various synthetic reactions.

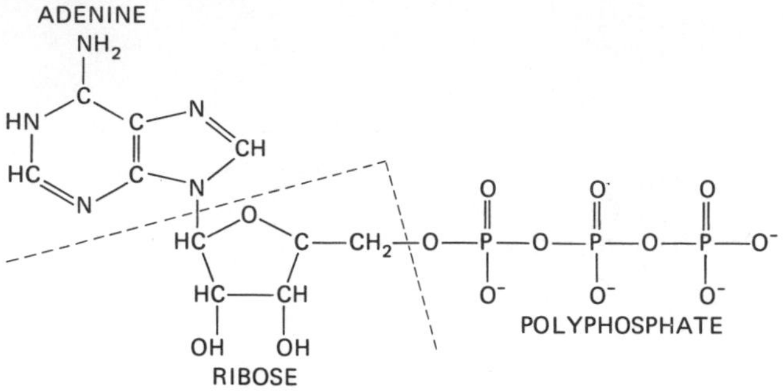

FIGURE II–4. The chemical formula of adenosine triphosphate (ATP). The molecule consists of a purine base adenine, the five-carbon sugar ribose, and three-phosphoric acid residues bonded together.

When these high-energy phosphate compounds are hydrolyzed in a calorimeter, they yield a large amount of energy in the form of heat. About 8,000 calories per mole are released when the terminal phosphate group of ATP is split off to form adenosine diphosphate (ADP). This value, expressed as $\Delta F = -8$ kcal/mole, represents the difference between the free energy of the reactant (ATP) and the product (ADP). Most low-energy phosphate compounds yield less than half this amount of heat when their bonds are split.

Cells control the release of energy, making it available as needed for functional processes. The reaction $ATP \rightleftharpoons ADP + P_i$ ($\Delta F = -8$ kcal /mole) plays a central role in this control process, since it allows energy-yielding reactions to be coupled with those requiring energy. The enzyme adenosine triphosphatase (ATPase) catalyzes the reaction.

A skeletal muscle cell provides an example of how this reaction is involved in the process of contraction (Fig. II–5). Two types of filaments, actin and myosin, are contained within the cytoplasm of the muscle cell. Their relationship to one another is responsible for the periodic cross-striations which appear as bands running across each myofibril (a bundle of myofilaments). One theory advanced to explain the contraction of a muscle cell involves the sliding of myosin with respect to actin (see Chapter VII). Mitochondria lie close to the myofibrils within the cytoplasm and they play an important role in supplying energy for this mechanical process.

Consider the following events as being part of the contraction process. An excitatory impulse travels along the membrane of the muscle cell and continues into deep invaginations of the cell membrane that are known as the transverse tubules (*T*-tubules). This excitatory stimulus causes calcium ions to be released (presumably from the sarcoplasmic reticulum) into the area of the myofibrils, where they activate myosin ATPase. As a result of myosin ATPase activity, inorganic phosphate (P_i) is split from ATP, and ADP is formed. With the energy released in this reaction, actin and myosin filaments, arranged in a parallel array, increase their interdigitations with respect to one another. The ADP then enters mitochondria where it acts as a phosphate acceptor. If there is enough oxidizable substrate available, the reverse of the above reaction occurs, and ADP becomes phosphorylated to ATP. Upon being released from mitochondria, the ATP is again available for the next cycle of contraction.

GLYCOLYSIS

The reactions of glycolysis occur outside mitochondria, within the cyto-plasm of the cell.[1] Molecular oxygen plays no role in this major metabolic pathway, which converts a single six-carbon glucose molecule into two three-carbon molecules, either pyruvate or lactate (Fig. II–6). Two phosphorylation reactions occur in this process and each one requires an ATP molecule. However, from each glucose four ATPs are formed, resulting in a net gain of two ATP molecules. (If the orginal compound to be broken down is glycogen, one ATP-requiring reaction is bypassed, so there is a net gain of three ATP molecules.) The change in free energy in the reaction

$$\text{glucose} \longrightarrow 2 \text{ lactic acid}$$

is -56 kcal/mole, slightly less than 10 percent of the potential energy contained in glucose (-680 kcal/mole). Glycolysis is an important pathway used by red blood cells, embryonic tissues, and cancer cells. Skeletal muscle also depends upon these reactions as a major source of energy.

An important link exists between the anaerobic reactions of glycolysis and the Krebs tricarboxylic acid cycle (discussed shortly). In the presence of oxygen, the pyruvic acid end product of glycolysis can enter the TCA cycle after being decarboxylated and converted into acetyl CoA. In this way the cell increases the efficiency of trapping the potential energy from the breakdown of glucose, as it burns the glucose completely to form carbon dioxide and water.

OXIDATIVE PHOSPHORYLATION

The oxidation of substrate in the presence of oxygen to form ATP is known as *oxidative phosphorylation*. It occurs within the mitochondria of cells and utilizes both the enzymes of the Krebs tricarboxylic acid cycle (TCA cycle) and those of the electron transport system (also known as the respiratory chain).

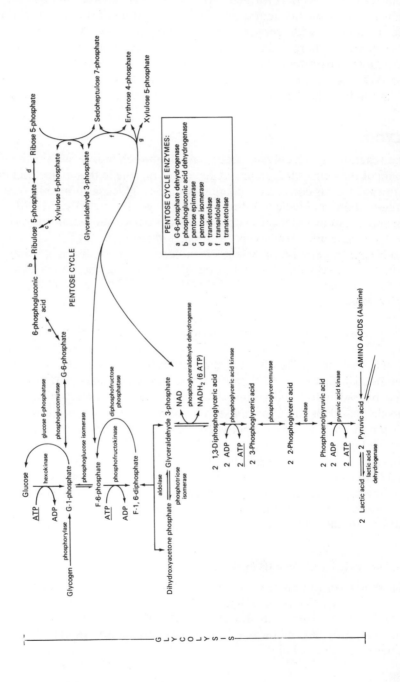

24

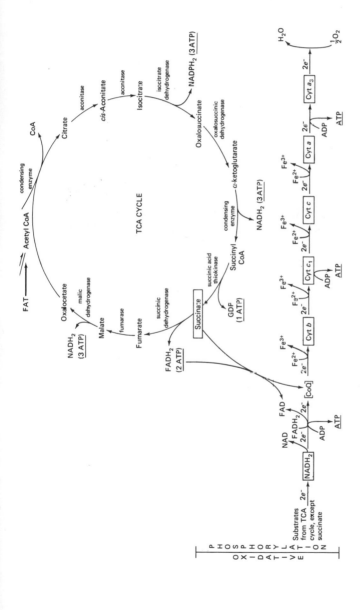

FIGURE II-6. Intermediary metabolism showing several pathways of energy production including glycolysis, pentose shunt, TCA cycle, and oxidative phosphorylation. The first two of these processes take place in the cell cytoplasm, the latter two in mitochondria.

KREBS TRICARBOXYLIC ACID CYCLE (TCA CYCLE)

Within the matrix of mitochondria the energy-producing reactions of the Krebs tricarboxylic acid cycle take place.[6] This cycle is a final central pathway for the degradation of carbohydrates, fats, and proteins. Metabolites are oxidized aerobically in this chain of reactions to yield carbon dioxide and water (Fig. II–6).

The first step in the cycle is the condensation of a two-carbon acetyl CoA molecule with oxaloacetic acid, a four-carbon compound to form the six-carbon citric acid molecule. In the sequence of reactions which follow, carbon dioxide is removed twice from the oxaloacetate residue. One complete turn of the cycle regenerates oxaloacetic acid which can again condense with acetyl CoA to form citric acid and thus begin another cycle.

ELECTRON TRANSPORT CHAIN

The Krebs tricarboxylic acid cycle is normally coupled to the electron transport chain. Certain substances such as dinitrophenol cause uncoupling of phosphorylation. When uncoupled respiration proceeds, electrons are transferred along the electron transport chain, but no ATP is formed.

In the reactions of glycolysis and the Krebs tricarboxylic acid cycle, hydrogen is removed from certain intermediate products in the presence of the carrier molecule *nicotinamide adenine dinucleotide* (NAD). NAD is a coenzyme required for the activity of certain enzymes. It accepts the hydrogen from an intermediate compound, which becomes oxidized, while NAD is reduced to $NADH_2$. In the course of these dehydrogenation reactions, the protons (H^+) and the electrons are separated and pass along the series of respiratory enzymes. This electron transport chain consists of yellow flavoproteins and red cytochromes. The cytochromes contain iron, which exists as Fe^{2+} in the reduced form. With the successive transfer of electrons, the reduced iron (Fe^{2+}) in the cytochromes is oxidized to the Fe^{3+} form. At the end of the electron transport chain the protons and electrons combine with oxygen to form water (Fig II–6). In three places along the chain, the energy of the oxidation–reduction process is used to regenerate ATP from inorganic phosphate and ADP.

In the processes of cell metabolism, wherever NAD captures hydrogen to form $NADH_2$, protons and electrons can be fed into the electron transport chain. Each $NADH_2$ therefore represents three potential ATP molecules (since there are three phosphorylation reactions in the chain) for each atom of oxygen reduced to water. The metabolite succinate feeds into the electron transport chain at coenzyme Q and thus bypasses one NAD step. Therefore, only two ATP molecules are formed in succinate oxidation for every atom of oxygen reduced (Fig II–6).

FATTY ACID OXIDATION

The Krebs tricarboxylic acid cycle is also linked to the metabolism of fats. Acetyl CoA is a major end product of fatty acid oxidation (also known as β-oxidation). The reactions involved in the breakdown of fatty acids also occur within mitochondria. Some time after a meal, or in starvation, when glucose and carbohydrates are in low supply, long-chained fatty acids (containing fourteen to twenty carbon atoms) furnish acetyl CoA to the TCA cycle. Fats actually provide more energy in the form of ATP than do carbohydrates. For each two-carbon acetyl CoA unit that is cleaved from a long-chained fatty acid (reactions not shown) during fatty acid oxidation (reactions not shown), five ATPs are formed. For example, palmitic acid (with sixteen carbon atoms) is degraded into eight acetyl CoA molecules after passing seven times through the reactions of β-oxidation (thus yielding 35 ATPs). Each of these eight acetyl CoAs will subsequently produce twelve more ATPs as they pass through the Krebs TCA cycle. β-oxidation of free fatty acids is the primary source of energy used by heart muscle.

PROTEIN AND AMINO ACID CATABOLISM

Proteins are broken down into amino acids by proteases. This enzymatic degradation occurs either extracellularly or within cytoplasmic lysosomes. The amino acids also form substrates for the Krebs tricarboxylic acid cycle by transferring their amine groups in a *transamination* reaction (Fig. II–7). As indicated, alanine is transaminated to pyruvic acid, which in turn is oxidized to acetyl CoA and carbon dioxide (CO_2). Glutamic acid often undergoes transamination to α-ketoglutaric acid, and aspartic acid enters the TCA cycle after being transaminated to oxaloacetic acid.

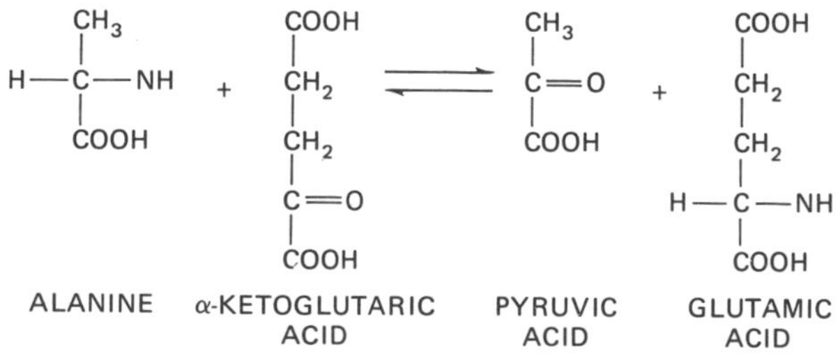

FIGURE II–7. A typical transamination reaction in which alanine is transaminated to pyruvic acid.

HEXOSE MONOPHOSPHATE SHUNT (PENTOSE CYCLE)

An alternative pathway of great significance in carbohydrate metabolism is the hexose monophosphate shunt (pentose cycle) (Fig.II–6). It occurs outside mitochondria and includes both an aerobic and an anaerobic pathway. From glucose 6-phosphate, an intermediate in glycolysis, two separate routes lead to the formation of ribose 5-phosphate. *Ribose* is a five-carbon sugar essential for the synthesis of nuleic acids. It appears that two separate pathways exist to ensure the production of ribose in case one chain of reactions becomes blocked. The hexose monophosphate shunt also provides a source of reduced nicotinamide adenine dinucleotide monophosphate ($NADPH_2$) needed for the synthesis of fatty acids and steroids. Although the pentose shunt pathway has not been demonstrated to be as widespread in cells as glycolysis, it is important in white blood cells, liver, and steroid-synthesizing tissues (for example, the adrenal cortex, testes, and so forth).

ENERGY YIELD AND EFFICIENCY

For each glucose molecule entering the TCA cycle, about thirty ATPs are formed, in contrast to glycolysis where either two or three ATPs are formed. Oxidative phosphorylation therefore produces ten to fifteen times more chemical energy than does anaerobic glycolysis. Cells show about a 50 percent efficiency in their production of energy, the remaining 50 percent being lost as heat (Table II–1).

METABOLIC REGULATION

Many metabolites in the cell can follow a variety of metabolic pathways. A good example of one such substance is glucose 6-phosphate. Its ultimate fate depends upon the particular needs of the animal. There are a number of potential routes it can follow: (1) it may be hydrolyzed in the presence of water to replenish the blood supply of glucose; (2) by forming glucose 1-phosphate, it may be used in the synthesis of liver glycogen; (3) transformed to ribose 5-phosphate, it becomes an important source of sugar for nucleic acid synthesis; (4) via breakdown during glycolysis and the TCA cycle, it furnishes energy; and (5) it can provide intermediates for the synthesis of fats and proteins.

The factors controlling regulation of cellular metabolism are under intense investigation. Some of the mechanisms responsible for determining which pathway an intermediate follows are being discovered. Hormones and certain metabolites have been found to influence particular reactions and thus designate which pathway is utilized.

TABLE II-1

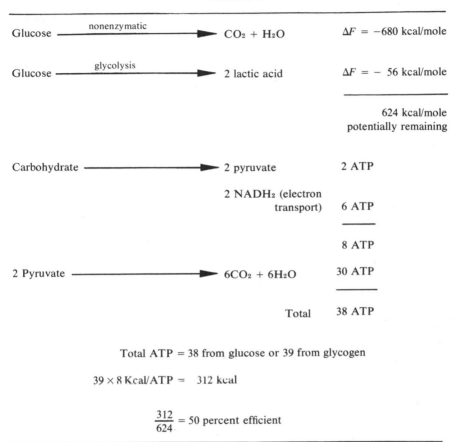

Glucose $\xrightarrow{\text{nonenzymatic}}$ $CO_2 + H_2O$		$\Delta F = -680$ kcal/mole
Glucose $\xrightarrow{\text{glycolysis}}$ 2 lactic acid		$\Delta F = -\ 56$ kcal/mole
		624 kcal/mole potentially remaining
Carbohydrate $\longrightarrow$ 2 pyruvate		2 ATP
	2 NADH$_2$ (electron transport)	6 ATP
		8 ATP
2 Pyruvate $\longrightarrow$ 6CO$_2$ + 6H$_2$O		30 ATP
	Total	38 ATP

Total ATP = 38 from glucose or 39 from glycogen

39×8 Kcal/ATP = 312 kcal

$$\frac{312}{624} = 50 \text{ percent efficient}$$

An important hypothesis explaining enzymatic control has recently been advanced. It is based upon the structure of regulatory enzymes and is known as *allosteric control*. As described earlier in this chapter, most enzyme–substrate reactions plot experimentally as hyperbolic curves. However, regulatory enzymes do not follow this pattern and their reactions with substrate molecules reveal S-shaped (sigmoid) curves.[4,8] The sigmoidal effect is explained by the structure of the regulatory enzyme molecule.

As mentioned earlier in this chapter, many regulatory enzymes have quaternary structure, that is, they are polymers, composed of several (identical) monomer subunits. These enzymes have a definite structural axis of symmetry which is maintained in the course of their interaction with substrate molecules (either inhibitors or activators). Aspartate transcarbamylase is a regulatory enzyme that consists of four monomers.[5]

It has been found that one of its monomers binds the substrate (active site), while another binds an inhibitor (regulatory site). All four monomer subunits interact to make this enzyme active or less active. The interaction of enzyme subunits is responsible for regulation, and because the active site and the regulatory site are separated within the molecule, their effects are said to be allosteric, or indirect.

An allosteric protein model has been proposed to help explain regulatory changes that occur within enzyme molecules (Fig. II–8)[3,7] An enzyme may be considered to exist in a "relaxed" state when it binds a substrate (or activator molecule). Its interaction with an inhibitor results in a molecular transition to a "constrained" state. The shifting back and forth between these two states is thought to be responsible for regulatory changes. Because the enzyme maintains its axis of symmetry, there is cooperation between the monomers. This interaction helps to explain the experimental sigmoid curve. Once a substrate molecule is bound to a monomer, the enzyme molecule is altered in such a way as to favor the binding of additional substrate. The balance between the two conformational states is therefore tipped toward the relaxed state, and substrate and activators are quickly bound. This accounts for a steep rise, thus resulting in an experimentally plotted S-shaped curve. The presence of appropriate inhibitor molecules, whether from end products or added experimentally, can cause an antagonistic interaction of the monomers and would tend to favor a constrained state. This model emphasizes

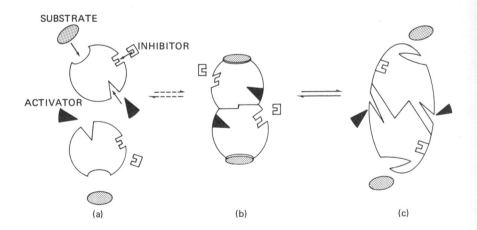

FIGURE II–8. Regulatory changes in an allosteric protein: (a) monomers; (b) polymer in "relaxed" state binds substrate and activator molecules; (c) polymer in "constrained" state binds inhibitors. Modified after J. P. Changeux, *Sci. Amer.* 212 (1965), 43.

the importance of structure at the molecular level. It postulates one mechanism of enzymatic control and regulation that depends entirely upon the conformation assumed by enzyme molecules.

REFERENCES

[1] Bernard Axelrod, "Glycolysis," in *Metabolic Pathways*, D. M. Greenberg, ed., Vol. I (New York: Academic Press Inc., 1960), 97–128.

[2] P. D. Boyer, Henry Lardy, and Karl Myrbäck, eds., *The Enzymes*, 2nd ed. (New York: Academic Press Inc., 1959).

[3] J. P. Changeux, "The Control of Biochemical Reactions," *Sci. Amer.*, 212 (1965), 36–45.

[4] J. S. Fruton and Sofia Simmonds, *General Biochemistry*, 2nd ed. (New York: John Wiley & Sons, Inc., 1958).

[5] J. C. Gerhart and A. B. Pardee, "Aspartate Transcarbamylase, an Enzyme Designed for Feedback Inhibition," *Fed. Proc.*, 23, 1 (1964), 727–735.

[6] H. A. Krebs and J. M. Lowenstein, "The Tricarboxylic Acid Cycle," in *Metabolic Pathways*, D. M. Greenberg, ed., Vol. 1 (New York: Academic Press Inc., 1960), 129–203.

[7] Jacques Monod, Jeffries Wyman, and J. P. Changeux, "On the Nature of Allosteric Transitions: A Plausible Model," *J. Mol. Biol.*, 12 (1965), 88–118.

[8] Abraham White, Philip Handler, and E. L. Smith, *Principles of Biochemistry,* 3rd ed. (New York: McGraw-Hill Book Co., 1964).

THE MACHINERY OF THE CYTOPLASM

CELLS

Living material is characterized by certain basic functions, including contractility, motility, reproduction, irritability, growth, respiration, adaptation, and metabolism. Living material is composed of cells and cell products. The cells are not only the fundamental unit of structure, but they are also the basic unit of these listed functions.

Since the cell was identified as the basic unit of life, scientists have been interested in learning how cells function. Throughout history, investigators have utilized the techniques available to them in order to discover more about the processes that comprise life. They have carefully observed cells under normal and experimental conditions, and recorded the responses of these minute structures when they are touched, injured, killed, or subjected to other experimental procedures.

With the perfected light microscope, scientists carefully observed cells in their living state and in fixed preparations. Many organs and tissue types were scrutinized and careful records were made of what was learned from the myriad of morphological patterns assumed by cells.

TISSUES AND ORGANS

Animal cells were seen to be associated in various patterns to form tissue. Four basic types of tissue have been identified: epithelial, connective, muscle, and nerve tissue.

Epithelial tissue is formed by cells which are closely attached to one another. Such sheets of epithelium line body surfaces and cavities and form glands.

In *connective tissue*, the cells are often widely dispersed in an abundant extracellular material. This extracellular material may be fluid (as in blood), semisolid (as in loose areolar connective tissue), firm (as in cartilage), or hard (as in bone).

Some cells contain large numbers of filaments which interact in such a way that they cause cell contraction and are called *muscle tissue*. When the filaments are in a highly ordered parallel array, the muscle cell takes on a striated appearance and is therefore called *striated* muscle. In some muscle cells, called *smooth* muscle, the filaments are not seen in as regular a manner and the cells do not contain striations.

Neurons are cells specialized for responding to external stimuli and transmitting nerve impulses. Along with other supportive and nutritive cells they comprise *nerve tissue*.

These four basic tissue types are associated in specific ways to form organs. For example, the wall of the intestine is made up of components of each tissue type. Lining the luminal surface of the intestine is a layer of columnar epithelial cells. The cells are closely attached. Some surface cells are involved in the absorption of substances formed in the breakdown of food products; others secrete mucus for lubrication of the luminal surface. The surface epithelium extends deep into the intestinal wall, forming glands which secrete various substances such as mucus and certain digestive enzymes.

The epithelium gains support from the connective tissue which underlies it. The connective tissue forms a layer of tissue containing the glands and also binds the epithelium to a deeper muscle layer. This muscle layer consists of a circularly oriented and a longitudinally oriented smooth muscle lamina. The contraction of these two laminae of muscle serve to mix and propel the food products within the digestive tract. Partial control of this muscle contraction comes from nerve cells and nerve cell processes which exist within these layers.

Blood vessels (another organ) penetrate the intestinal wall. These vessels in turn are made up of endothelium (a type of epithelium), connective tissue, and muscle. Moreover the muscle contraction is controlled by nerve cell processes.

In turn, individual organs are associated to form organ systems such as the digestive system, circulatory system, and respiratory system.

The development of the electron microscope, with its increased resolving power, stimulated a new effort to describe the internal machinery of these various types of cells. Since then, there has been a productive period in which scientists have described the internal structure of a variety of cell types under many different physiological conditions. It has become evident that many organelles are found in most cells studied (Fig. III–1). Once this cellular machinery had been described, interest shifted to elucidating how it worked. Techniques such as autoradiography, histochemistry, cell fractionation, and biochemical determinations, which were described briefly in Chapter I, have been applied to normal and experimentally altered tissue in an effort to achieve this goal. The study of unusual biological specializations which have resulted from the complex evolutionary process, such as the nasal salt-excreting glands of marine birds, is also being used by scientists to contribute additional knowledge in this area. Some pertinent information about the major functional machinery of the cytoplasm is presented in this chaper.

PROCARYOTIC AND EUCARYOTIC CELLS

This book deals almost exclusively with *eucaryotic* animal cells and, more specifically, with cells from vertebrates. Eucaryotic cells are to be distinguished from *procaryotic* cells, which are apparently more primitive and are found only among the bacteria and blue-green algae. There are major structural and biochemical differences between procaryotes and eucaryotes. Perhaps the most important difference is that in procaryotes the genome is found naked in the cytoplasm, while in eucaryotes the typical mitotic chromosomes and interphase nucleus, surrounded by a nuclear membrane, are present. Procaryotic cells also have no mitochondria or plastids, while eucaryotic cells nearly always possess these organelles. Nevertheless, there are features in common to both eucaryotic and procaryotic cells. These include (1) the presence of a cell membrane as a selective permeability barrier and (2) the presence of major central biochemical pathways including a replicating genome of DNA and protein synthesis on ribosomes.

There are also major differences between eucaryotic animal and plant cells. The presence of a rigid cell wall around plant cells has far-reaching consequences because plants tend to use osmotic devices for growth or responses to stimuli. Usually plant cells contain *chloroplasts* or other plastids which are capable of photosynthesis. Many plants have lost the centrioles and centriolar derivatives, while the centriole is a typical animal organelle involved in mitosis (although it is lost in amoebae). However, most of the organelles discussed in this chapter are present in all eucaryotic cells whether plant or animal. These include the cell membrane, the nucleus, the mitochondria, the endoplasmic reticulum, the ribosomes, the Golgi apparatus, and related membrane systems.

CELL MEMBRANE AND THE UNIT MEMBRANE CONCEPT

The existence of a cell membrane was first surmised from a variety of observations, including the following: (1) cells have the ability to shrink and swell depending upon the tonicity of their surrounding medium; (2) cell boundaries can arrest the movement of dye injected into the cell; and (3) a subsequent loss of cell contents occurs when the surface is disrupted by any one of a number of procedures.[4] The cell membrane serves not only to enclose the cell and partially to protect it from hostile environmental conditions but also to house the biochemical mechanisms which are involved in providing energy for the transport of certain substances into and out of the cell.

Isolated cell membranes are readily obtained from mammalian red blood cells. The red cells, which consist of the protein hemoglobin surrounded by a cell membrane, are lysed by being placed in *hypotonic* solutions. Water is drawn into the cells by osmosis, causing an initial swelling. A change in membrane permeability results and hemoglobin escapes, presumably leaving only the cell membrane. When the lipid content of lysed red blood cell membranes was measured, enough lipid was found to form a double layer of lipid molecules each 30 to 40 Ångström units thick over the entire cell surface.[11] The presence of a double-layered lipid structure is consistent with the observed high permeability of the cell membrane to lipid-soluble substances and low permeability to the passage of certain ionic materials which are lipid insoluble. In order to explain various other physical properties demonstrated by cell membranes, such as low surface tension, it was postulated that the thin continuous bimolecular lipid layer was oriented so that the hydrophilic polar groups of the lipid molecules were on the outside and a layer of denatured protein molecules could be adsorbed on the two polar surfaces of the membrane.[6] It has also been proposed that a further layer of globular proteins coats the denatured protein layer.[6]

When cells are fixed and prepared for electron microscopy, a thin dense layer is seen at the interface between the cell and the surrounding medium. In many instances, this layer can be resolved to contain three constituent sublayers consisting of two dense lines 20 to 30 Ångström units wide separated by an intervening light area approximately 35 Ångström units in width (Fig. III–2). Because this triple-layered structure is so frequently seen, it has been termed the *unit membrane*.[32] Each of the dense lines is thought to represent the polar ends of the lipid molecules together with the adsorbed surface coat of protein. The unit membrane differs somewhat in its appearance from cell to cell. In fact, thickness and density of three sublayers can vary depending upon the type of tissue being studied and the technique of preparation used. Different membranes share wide variations in chemical composition as well. Animal cell membranes contain complex mixtures of phosphatides, whereas certain bacterial membranes contain only phosphatidyl ethanolamine. Cholesterol is found in animal membranes but not in bacterial membranes.[40] This may reflect basic biochemical differences in eucaryotic versus procaryotic cells. Membranes also exist within the cell and the thickness of some of these membranes differs from those seen surrounding the cell.[36,42]

Although many biologists believe that the unit membrane seen in electron micrographs represents the structure of the unaltered membrane which exists around living cells, other hypotheses for the structure of cell membranes in the living state have been proposed. One such alternative hypothesis suggests that certain membranes might be composed of a layer of globular structures which represent lipid *micelles,* coated on both internal and external surfaces of the globule layer with a thin layer of protein.[10,17] A third hypothesis states that some membranes are composed of lipid globules coated with proteins and suggests in addition that protein septa also exist as bridges between the micellar subunits.[35,36]

Recent studies indicate that much of the membrane protein is in the globular α-helical conformation and not extended in the β-conformation. The accumulation of such chemical and spectroscopic evidence, which does not fit with the more traditional ideas discussed above, has led to the formation of new models which demonstrate more closely the fact that α-protein forms an integral part of the membrane in living cells.[40]

Since enzymes involved in ion transport form part of the cell membrane, further studies of the enzymatic activity of various cell membranes and of model membrane systems that transport ions will contribute to our knowledge of membrane structure. In a similar manner, since preparatory procedures may affect the true structure of the membrane, what we learn about the alteration which can occur during these procedures may help us to obtain a clearer picture of the membrane structure *in vivo.*

Although all membranes have some properties in common, certain membranes have specialized activities. Presumably, therefore, the enzymatic makeup of specific membranes may also vary. The membrane surrounding the cell differs enzymatically from membranes found within the cell. Moreover, membranes are dynamic structures and may not always be in the same state of activity during life. It is conceivable that their structure might change in accordance with fluctuations or shifts in their activity.

Besides variations within the membranes themselves, a variety of specialized areas are found along the outer membranes of cells. These are involved in the maintenance of cell shape, the uptake of material, shunts of low electrical resistance, and cell-to-cell adhesion. These membrane modifications are discussed in detail in subsequent chapters.

NUCLEUS

In eucaryotic cells, the nucleus is usually distinguished from the cytoplasm per se. Its morphology is discussed briefly here because of the important influence it exerts upon the working cytoplasm. The nucleus plays a role similar to that of the executive office of a factory: (1) The nucleus contains the genetic material (the blueprint) which was used in the construction of the cell, and which, in turn, can replicate to produce other cells; and (2) the nucleus appears to control the metabolic activity of the cell by producing a long strand of coded information (the production order) called *messenger ribonucleic acid* (mRNA). This coded directive has been shown to move from the nucleus into the cytoplasm, perhaps through the cylindrical channels called *nuclear pores* (Fig. III–3), which penetrate the *nuclear envelope*.

The genetic material in eucaryotic cells is arranged at specific sites (genes) in a linear sequence along *chromosomes*. The chromosomes are found in the chromatin regions of the nucleus and they have been shown to have a high content of *deoxyribonucleic acid* (DNA). *Chromatin* exists in two states. The condensed areas of chromatin stain more intensely and have been called *heterochromatin*; the less condensed areas, which presumably contain a more dispersed form of DNA, are called *euchromatin* (Fig. III–3). Euchromatin predominates when the cell is metabolically active. During cell division, all areas of chromatin are condensed to form visible chromosomes (Fig. III–4).[9]

One or more *nucleoli* are found in the nucleus (Fig. III–5). Nucleoli vary in size and shape, being well developed when the cytoplasm is involved in active synthetic processes and disappearing during division. Several lines of evidence implicate nucleoli in the production of *ribosomal ribonucleic acid* (rRNA) that is utilized in the synthesis of protein in the cytoplasm. Morphologically, nucleoli consist of two main components (Fig. III–5): (1) a twisted thread-like structure called the *nucleolenema* which is composed of fibrillar regions and contains granules measuring approximately 150 Ångström units in diameter; and (2) compact finely granular areas called the *pars amorpha*.[9] The nucleolenema presumable is composed of precursor molecules of ribosomal RNA. These precursor molecules give rise to both the subunits of the ribosome.

In eucaryotic cells, the nucleus is separated from the cytoplasm by the nuclear envelope (Fig. III–3). In procaryotes, a nuclear region can be identified, but, as we already noted, there is no nuclear envelope.[3] The nuclear envelope is similar in appearance to parts of the endoplasmic reticulum to which it is frequently attached and from which it may be derived (or which may be derived from it). The envelope consists of two unit membranes, each approximately 75 Ångström units wide, containing a space between them called the *perinuclear cisterna*. A large number of cylinders of approximately 500 Ångström units in diameter, called nuclear pores, penetrate the nuclear envelope. These appear to form by the fusion of the two membranes composing the nuclear envelope and the obliteration of the perinuclear cisterna. A thin layer of material that may act as a diaphragm is frequently seen bridging the circular gap of the nuclear pore.[41] It is presumed that some material passes from nucleus to cytoplasm and vice versa through the nuclear pores.

RIBOSOMES AND POLYSOMES

Granules approximately 150 to 200 Ångström units in diameter are found within the cytoplasm of all cells that synthesize proteins. These granules, called *ribosomes,* are rich in ribonucleic acid and protein. Each ribosome is composed of two subunits of unequal size which have specific functions in protein synthesis (see Chapter V). Ribosomes are frequently found in clusters or patterned arrays which have been called *polysomes.* In bacterial cells polysomes have been shown to be held together by their relationship to mRNA. Ribosomes are frequently seen free in the cytoplasm of cells which are active in synthesizing protein for intracellular use. In cells which synthesize protein for export, the granules are found in whorls or rows along the cytoplasmic surface of certain intracellular membranes called endoplasmic reticulum.

ENDOPLASMIC RETICULUM

Before techniques were developed for tissue sectioning, electron microscopists could only examine thin cell layers. Cells grown in tissue culture that had thin regions near their peripheries were studied. A network (or reticulum) was seen permeating the entire cytoplasm of these cells except at their most peripheral zone (ectoplasmic layer). Therefore, Porter and his associates[27,28,30] referred to this network as the *endoplasmic reticulum* and suggested that it corresponded to areas of the cytoplasm that stained intensely with basic dyes (ergastoplasm). In thin sections it became evident that the endoplasmic reticulum was a vast network composed of large flattened membrane-bound areas of cisternae, tubules, and vesicles of various shapes and sizes. This extensive reticulum can thus be viewed as a large, potentially intercommunicating system, at times continuous with the nuclear membrane.[12]

The membranes of the endoplasmic reticulum vary in amount and in their enzymatic content, depending upon the type of cell and upon its stage of development. The form of the endoplasmic reticulum may be altered in many ways, including its response to various cell injuries.

Two types of endoplasmic reticulum have been identified.[9] The first type is called *rough-surfaced endoplasmic reticulum* (granular endoplasmic reticulum), because the cytoplasmic surfaces of the membranes are studded with adherent ribosomes (Fig. III–6). The granular endoplasmic reticulum reaches its greatest development in cells specialized to make protein products to be secreted from the cell, in, for example, exocrine cells of the pancreas (see Chapter V).[2] In these cells, multiple layers of cisternae fill most of the cytoplasm. If the membranes and cisternae of the endoplasmic reticulum are considered an assembly line, the attached ribosomes are analogous to the workers because they participate in the assembly of proteins. As they are being made, the proteins cross the membrane and are transported within the cisternal space of the endoplasmic reticulum.

The second type of endoplasmic reticulum is called the *smooth-surfaced endoplasmic reticulum* (agranular endoplasmic reticulum) (Fig. III–7). The smooth-surfaced endoplasmic reticulum appears to be a system of interconnected tubules and is found in abundance in many cell types. Cells which are known to be producing steroids and related compounds frequently exhibit highly developed agranular endoplasmic reticulum, which presumably plays a role in the biosynthesis of these compounds.[5] Liver cells respond to the administration of lipid-soluble drugs by increasing their content of agranular endoplasmic reticulum. There is also an associated increase in the enzymes which metabolize or detoxify the administered drugs.[29] Presumably, these enzymes are located in the newly formed membranes. In other cells, the agranular endoplasmic reticulum appears to be associated with the resynthesis of triglycerides. Smooth-surfaced endoplasmic reticulum appears to play some role in the metabolism of glycogen because of its frequent association with areas of the cytoplasm which are richly endowed with particles of glycogen.[9] Although smooth-surfaced endoplasmic reticulum exhibits a similar appearance in each of these cells, it is likely that the enzymatic content of its membrane differs in relation to its function.

The width of the agranular endoplasmic reticulum membrane usually measures approximately 50 Ångström units.[36] However, in certain ion-transporting cells the membranes of this organelle appear to be thicker and are frequently seen communicating with the cell membrane. This thicker membrane is found in cells involved either in the secretion of hydrochloric acid, as in the stomach,[16] or in the transcellular transport of chloride ion, as in the teleost gill.[26] This type of agranular endoplasmic reticulum can be distinguished morphologically. Perhaps when more is learned about the precise biochemical functions of cell membranes, further morphological subtypes of smooth-surfaced endoplasmic reticulum will be recognized.

MITOCHONDRIA

The cell requires energy in order to maintain its ionic equilibrium under resting conditions as well as to accomplish specific metabolic goals. Glycogen particles and fat droplets, which are visible on electron micrographs, as well as a number of smaller molecules such as glucose, which are too small to be resolved at the present time by the electron microscope, are oxidized by the cell to produce energy. Oxidative energy is released from these compounds, by oxidative phosphorylation, and is stored for use in the compound adenosine triphosphate (ATP). The chief production of ATP in most cells occurs in a group of organelles called *mitochondria*. In living cells, the mitochondria move, divide, branch, fuse, and actively change shape. In electron micrographs of fixed cells, mitochondria assume a variety of shapes (Figs. III–8, III–9). These organelles consist of two membranes and the enclosed area. The *inner membrane* often is thrown into thin folds which penetrate the central cavity of the mitochondrion. These folds are called *cristae mitochondriales* and form incomplete (or occasionally complete) septa dividing the central cavity. The space between the internal and external membranes of the mitochondrion and the space inside of the cristae mitochondriales is known as the *intracristal space*. The space internal to the inner membrane of the mitochondria is known as the *matrix*. Dense granules approximately 300 to 1,000 Ångström units in diameter can be seen within the matrix.[24]

The exact configuration of the cristae of mitochondria varies, depending upon the type of cell and its state of metabolic activity. The cristae can appear as tubules, honeycombed membranes, membranes with angulations, or sheets of membranes.[31]

If mitochondria are broken open and the membranes negatively stained by immersing them in an extremely electron-dense substance, the inner membrane displays small subunits along its surface. The exact nature of these particles is not known, but some workers believe that these subunits contain an enzyme called F_1 which has ATPase activity.[23] Whether these surface subunits are present in the *in vivo* mitochondrion or are created by the experimental procedure has been questioned.[37]

Mitochondria also have been shown to contain other substances.[15] Molecules of DNA in the form of a double helix have been identified within mitochondria.[18,19] In some cases the DNA is in a circular form similar to that found in bacteria. Mitochondrial ribosomes are also thought to be present. This synthetic system is presently thought to be concerned with replication of certain mitochondrial proteins. The genes for synthesis of other prominent parts of the electron transport system are nuclear genes, however. The exact process by which mitochondria replicate their membrane elements is still unknown.

Mitochondria frequently are located adjacent to cell membranes, muscle fibers, lipid droplets, or cisternae of the endoplasmic reticulum, where chemical reactions and/or active transport occur.

CHLOROPLASTS AND OTHER PLASTIDS

The presence of *plastids* is a distinguishing characteristic of plant cells. The most common type of plastid is a *chloroplast,* which contains chlorophyll pigments (Fig. III–10). These chlorophyll pigments allow the capturing of the light energy from the sun and the conversion of it into chemical energy that can be utilized by the cell. The chlorophyll pigment is part of a membrane system of the plastid just as the membranes of the mitochondria house some of the components of the electron transport chain. In higher plants, the internal membranes of a chloroplast are complex. The chlorophyll pigment is found in the fused stacks of flattened discs called *grana*. Additional membrane sheets connect the grana. Chloroplasts have also been shown to contain DNA and ribosomes.

GOLGI APPARATUS

The *Golgi apparatus* is the site at which most synthesized proteins appear to be condensed and packaged for secretion. Recent evidence indicates that it is also one site at which glycoproteins and mucopolysaccharides are synthesized and added to the protein to be secreted.[20,21] The Golgi apparatus consists of three kinds of membrane-bound structures (Fig. III–11). First there are cup-shaped stacks of flattened sacs, or cisternae, piled in roughly parallel array.[9] Within these cisternae is a cavity that in most areas measures approximately 150 Ångström units across; the layers of membranes appear to be spaced approximately 200 to 300 Ångström units apart. These cisternae are, however, more closely spaced than the parallel arrays of membranes comprising the endoplasmic reticulum. However, localized areas of the cisternae are frequently dilated to form saccules. The second Golgi component consists of vesicles which surround the membrane stacks and range in size from 400 to 800 Ångström units in diameter. The membranes of these vesicles may be coated on their cytoplasmic side with a layer of material or they may be entirely smooth surfaced.[9] The third component of the Golgi apparatus consists of vacuoles, which are seen most frequently in cells involved in the secretion of certain protein products. The vacuoles are often spherical, and found in close association with the other two elements of the Golgi apparatus. The vacuoles may appear empty or may contain material of varying density. The material sometimes resembles that within the secretion granules also present in the particular cell being examined.

Cells involved in secretion appear to have well-developed Golgi areas. In fact, many such cells display several separate Golgi profiles which appear to outline a cytoplasmic zone or form a cap over the nucleus.

Recent experiments indicate that the Golgi apparatus may also function in the synthesis of certain products, such as mucosubstances. Radioactive glucose has been injected into rats and their colons removed at measured time intervals after administration of this sugar.[21] At 5 minutes the label was incorporated into substances within saccules of the Golgi. At later time points, the label was seen over the mucous granules. Therefore, it appears that complex carbohydrates form within the Golgi region itself.[20,21,25]

The cellular product which is packaged and condensed in the Golgi region can either be stored within the cytoplasm for varying periods of time, or it can move to the periphery of the cell for subsequent release. Release of a product by a cell involves fusion of the packaging membrane with the surface membrane of the cell. Following this fusion, the free product, devoid of its packaging membrane, is released. As a result of this membrane fusion during release of a product, the Golgi apparatus becomes a source for the replacement of the surface cell membrane. The cell membrane which is derived from the Golgi apparatus in this manner appears to replace membrane used up in other processes such as phagocytosis. Bennett[1] proposed the concept that the membranes of the cell are in a continuous dynamic state of flow. According to this hypothesis, membrane taken into the cell during the uptake of various substances circulates as some intracellular membrane, and eventually is returned to the cell surface. The Golgi region appears to play an important role in this process. Its function may be to convert membranes from the intracellular type to the cell surface type, and/or to permit a substance lying in the lumen of a membrane-bound channel to be moved from one type of packaging to another.

In some epithelial cells the membranes of the Golgi cisternae and those of the endoplasmic reticulum are of a thinner type than those of the Golgi vesicles and the surface cell membrane.[42] In general, it is thought that thin-type membranes do not fuse with thick-type membranes. However, an exception to this rule may be found in the Golgi apparatus, where both membrane types exist. In the Golgi area, material surrounded by thin membranes (from the endoplasmic reticulum) appears to be transferred into secretory granules bound by thick membranes. These granules may in turn fuse with the surface cell membrane, allowing for the release of the contained product.

PHAGOSOME–LYSOSOME SYSTEM

Raw materials to be used by the cell can come from a source external (exogenous) to the cell. Some small molecules can gain entrance by directly penetrating cell membranes. Larger materials from an external source are taken up by entering into invaginating membrane-lined cavities of the surface membrane in a process called *endocytosis*. When the materials come from an external source, the endocytic uptake process is sometimes also called heterophagy.[7] The size of these raw materials ranges from small molecules to entire cells. The first step in the uptake of substances appears to be related to the binding of the material to some external coat of the cell membranes. The invaginating cavities pinch off, forming membrane-bound phagosomes. According to data from histochemical techniques, these phagosomes do not contain the hydrolytic enzymes involved in the breakdown of the various materials which have been sequestered. In these regions of invaginating membranes, the cytoplasmic surfaces show bristle-like or spiny projections.[33,34] After phagosomes are formed from the cell surface, they are able to migrate into the cell, where they fuse with certain other membrane-bounded components in the cytoplasm called *lysosomes* (Fig. III–12).[7]

Raw materials also can be derived from the sequestering of areas of the cell itself. In these cases the source is internal (endogenous) and the process of sequestering is called *autophagy*.[7] During this process, an area of the cytoplasm, and its organelles, appears to become enveloped by a flattened sac consisting of two membranes. The inner of these membranes disappears, leaving a single membrane-limited body. This process of sequestering can occur normally or, probably more often, as a reaction to sublethal injury.[39]

Heterophagic or autophagic vacuoles are converted into lysosomes by the addition of hydrolytic enzymes to the membrane-limited bodies.

Hydrolytic enzymes capable of breaking down all major types of molecules, including proteins, lipids, nucleic acids, and polysaccharides, have been identified within lysosomes.[7] Although much material appears to be digested for reutilization as cellular raw material, a certain amount of nondigested (residual) material appears to remain within these hydrolase-containing bags. The ultimate fate of this material is not always clear. However, in some cell populations which border on a lumen, lysosomes with large amounts of debris appear to migrate back to the cell surface to discharge their contents into the lumen.

Cells have adapted the processes of endocytosis and digestion not only for obtaining raw materials (as was the major use in unicellular organisms) but also to fulfill many other needs. It appears that such mechanisms operate in the defense against invading bacteria, for disposing of unused and unwanted cell organelles, and for the control of hormone production or secretion.[7] It has been shown that deficiencies of certain hydrolytic enzymes in lysosomes are associated with diseases. These processes are examined in detail in Chapter VII.

MICROBODIES (PEROXISOMES)

Microbodies are single-membrane-limited inclusions found in liver and kidney cells and in other tissue types. They have a moderately dense matrix, and in certain species contain a dense core-like structure (nucleoid), and/or plate-like structures called marginal plates.[8] Microbodies are partially surrounded by membranous cisternae of the endoplasmic reticulum (Fig. III–13). The origin of microbodies remains uncertain, although they may arise from and bud off the endoplasmic reticulum.[22]

Microbodies have been partly characterized biochemically and have been shown to contain catalase and oxidase enzymes.[8] Because these enzymes play a role in hydrogen peroxide metabolism, microbodies are also called peroxisomes.[8] It is thought that peroxisomes are active metabolic units involved in a special kind of respiration. This entire electron transfer process may be written

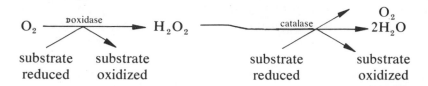

Oxidase enzymes first reduce oxygen to hydrogen peroxide at the same time as they are oxidizing a substrate. In a second phase of this respiration, hydrogen peroxide is reduced to water by the enzyme catalase. This second part of the respiratory process proceeds by two separate mechanisms: (1) either a substrate molecule acts as an electron donor; or (2) a second molecule of hydrogen peroxide serves this function. It is thought that the catalase in peroxisomes may act as a protective safety device, allowing for the disposal of excess hydrogen peroxide. If hydrogen peroxide accumulates in high amounts, it is harmful to cells.

Peroxisomes may also play a role in the synthesis of carbohydrates. Because they serve as a pathway for the formation of α-keto acids,[8] which are the main building blocks for carbohydrate synthesis, they might directly participatae in gluconeogenesis (the formation of glucose from noncarbohydrate precursors). Some cells in which peroxisomes are found have little ability to oxidize carbohydrates, but are primary sites for gluconeogenesis. In liver cells, peroxisomes are found to increase in number when animals are treated with drugs that lower plasma lipids.[13,38] This suggests that liver peroxisomes may be utilizing plasma lipids to synthesize glucose. Furthermore, peroxisome activity has been found in the protozoan *Tetrahymena pyriformis,* an organism known for its ability to synthesize carbohydrates from fat.[14] These findings are highly suggestive that peroxisomes play a role in carbohydrate synthesis.

Another possible function of peroxisomes is the oxidation of $NADH_2$ to NAD^+.[8] As $NADH_2$ is formed within the cytoplasmic matrix of the cell, peroxisomes would oxidize it and thus provide aerobic support for metabolic functions in the cytoplasm. Until recently this role has been attributed to mitochondria. The significance of peroxisomes and their role in various metabolic processes is only now being discovered.[8]

CENTRIOLES, SPINDLE FIBERS, AND MICROTUBULES

A pair of small cylindrical structures called centrioles are often seen in the juxtanuclear zone of cells. The cylinders are about 3,000 to 5,000 Ångström units in length and 1,500 Ångström units in diameter. The wall of the cylinder is composed of nine triplets of hollow tubules.[9] Although one can generally locate only a single pair of centrioles in a cell, the centrioles replicate before cell division occurs. During division a pair of centrioles is thereby found at either side of the nucleus. The spindle fibers (microtubules) which form during division converge upon the centrioles and terminate in dense satellites adjacent to the centriole.

In addition to the microtubules which form the spindle fibers during mitosis, additional microtubules within the cytoplasm of most cells has recently been appreciated. Microtubules are usually long straight or gently curving structures with an outside diameter of ~250 Ångström units and an electron-lucent center. Their function is discussed in Chapter IV. Microtubules that form centriolar walls, the main structure of cilia and flagella, spindle fibers, and other cell structures are related structures composed of proteins called *tubulin*. These proteins exist in an unpolymerized state in the cell cytoplasm until they are incorporated into the growing microtubule. Thus, microtubules are one cell component that can be assembled or disassembled at different points in the cell's lifetime. This accounts for the appearance and disappearance of the mitotic apparatus. Some microtubules, such as the spindle fibers, have relatively short lifetimes, while others, such as centriolar microtubules, are quite stable and persist for long periods of time.

REFERENCES

[1]H. Stanley Bennett, "The Concepts of Membrane Flow and Membrane Vesiculation as Mechanisms for Active Transport and Ion Pumping," *J. Biophys, Biochem. Cytol.*, Suppl. 2, 4 (1956), 99–103.

[2]L. G. Caro and G. E. Palade, "Protein Synthesis, Storage and Discharge in the Pancreatic Exocrine Cell. An Autoradiographic Study," *J. Cell Biol.*, 20 (1964), 473–495.

[3]L. G. Caro, P. van Tubergen, and Frederick Forro, Jr., "The Localization of Deoxyribonucleic Acid in *Escherichia Coli,*" *J. Biophys. Biochem. Cytol.*, 4 (1958), 491–494.

[4]Robert Chambers, "The Nature of the Living Cell as Revealed by Microdissection," *Harvey Lectures*, 22 (1926–1927), 41–58.

[5]A. Christensen and D. W. Fawcett, "The Normal Fine Structure of Opossum Testicular Interstitial Cells," *J. Biophys. Biochem. Cytol.*, 9 (1961), 653–670.

[6]J. F. Danielli and Hugh Davson, "A Contribution to the Theory of Permeability of Thin Films," *J. Cell. Comp. Physiol.*, 5 (1935), 495–508.

[7]Christian de Duve and Robert Wattiaux, "Functions of Lysosomes," *Ann. Rev. Physiol.*, 28 (1966), 435–492.

[8]Christian de Duve and Pierre Baudhuin, "Peroxisomes (Microbodies and Related Particles)," *Physiol. Rev.*, 46 (1966), 323–356.

[9]D. W. Fawcett, *An Atlas of Fine Structure. The Cell: Its Organelles and Inclusions* (Philadelphia: W. B. Saunders Co., 1966).

[10]A. M. Glauert, "Electron Microscopy of Lipids and Membranes," *J. Royal Microscop. Soc.*, 88 (1968), 49–70.

[11]E. Gorter and F. Grendel, "On Bimolecular Layers of Lipoids on the Chromocytes of the Blood," *J. Exp. Med.*, 41 (1925), 439–443.

[12] Francoise Haguenau, "The Ergastoplasm: Its History, Ultrastructure and Biochemistry," *Int. Rev. Cytol.*, 7 (1958), 425–483.

[13] R. Hess, W. Reiss, and W. Stäubli "Hepatic Actions of Hypolipidaemic Drugs: Effect of Ethyl Chlorophenoxyisobutyrate (CPIB)," in *Progress in Biochemical Pharmacology*, D. Kritchevsky, R. Paoletti, and D. Seinberg, eds., Vol. 2, Drugs Affecting Lipid Metabolism, Pt. 1, (Basal/New York: S. Kargger AG, 1967), 325–336.

[14] J. F. Hogg and H. L. Kornberg, "The Metabolism of C_2-Compounds in Micro-Organisms. 9. Role of the Glyoxylate Cycle in Protozoal Glyconeogenesis," *Biochem. J.*, 86 (1963), 462–468.

[15] A. L. Lehninger, "Molecular Basis of Mitochondrial Structure and Function," in *Molecular Organization and Biological Function*, J. M. Allen, ed. (New York, Harper & Row, Inc., 1967), pp. 107–133.

[16] C. B. Lillibridge, "Electron Microscopic Measurements of the Thickness of Various Membranes in Oxyntic Cells from Frog Stomach," *J. Ultrastruct. Res.*, 23 (1968), 243–259.

[17] J. A. Lucy and A. M. Glauert, "Structure and Assembly of Macromolecular Lipid Complexes Composed of Globular Micelles," *J. Mol. Biol.*, 8 (1964), 727–748.

[18] M. M. K. Nass and Sylvan Nass, "Intramitochondrial Fibers with DNA Characteristics. I. Fixation and Electron Staining Reactions," *J. Cell Biol.*, 19 (1963), 593–611.

[19] Sylvan Nass and M. M. K. Nass, "Intramitochondrial Fibers with DNA Characteristics. II. Enzymatic and Other Hydrolytic Treatments," *J. Cell Biol.*, 19 (1963), 613–629.

[20] Marian Neutra and C. P. Leblond, "Synthesis of the Carbohydrate of Mucus in the Golgi Complex as shown by Electron Microscope Radioautography of Goblet Cells from Rats Injected with Glucose-H³," *J. Cell Biol.*, 30 (1966), 119–136.

[21] Marian Neutra and C. P. Leblond, "Radioautographic Comparison of the Uptake of Galactose-H³ and Glucose-H³ in the Golgi Region of Various Cells Secreting Glycoproteins or Mucopolysaccharides," *J. Cell Biol.*, 30 (1966), 137–150.

[22] A. B. Novikoff and W. Y. Shin, "The Endoplasmic Reticulum in the Golgi Zone and Its Relations to Microbodies, Golgi Apparatus and Autophagic Vacuoles in Rat Liver Cells," *J. Microscopie*, 3 (1964), 187–206.

[23] D. F. Parsons, "Recent Advances Correlating Structure and Function in Mitochondria," in *Intern Rev. Exp. Path.*, G. W. Richter and M. A. Epstein, eds., Vol. 4 (New York: Academic Press Inc., 1965) 1–54.

[24] L. D. Peachey, "Electron Microscopic Observations on the Accumulation of Divalent Cations in Intramitochondrial Granules," *J. Cell Biol.*, 20 (1964), 95–111.

[25] Marian Peterson and C. P. Leblond, "Synthesis of Complex Carbohydrates in the Golgi Region, as Shown by Radioautography after Injection of Labeled Glucose," *J. Cell Biol.*, 21 (1964), 143–148.

[26] C. W. Philpott, "Electrolyte Transport and Acid Mucopolysaccharides of the Cell Surface," *J. Cell Biol.*, 23 (1964), 74A.

[27] K. R. Porter, "Observations on a Submicroscopic Basophilic Component of Cytoplasm," *J. Exp. Med.*, 97(1953), 727–750.

[28] K. R. Porter, "The Ground Substance; Observations from Electron Microscopy," in the *The Cell: Biochemistry, Physiology, Morphology,* Jean Brachet and A. E. Mirsky, eds., (New York: Academic Press Inc., 1961), Vol. 2, 621–675.

[29] K. R. Porter and Carlo Bruni, "An Electron Microscope Study of the Early Effects of 3-Me-DAB on Rat Liver Cells," *Cancer Res.*, 19 (1959), 997–1009.

[30] K. R. Porter, Albert Claude, and E. F. Fullam, "A Study of Tissue Culture Cells by Electron Microscopy. Methods and Preliminary Observations," *J. Exp. Med.*, 81 (1945), 233–246.

[31] J.-P. Revel, D. W. Fawcett, and C. W. Philpott, "Observations on Mitochondrial Structure. Angular Configurations of the Cristae," *J. Cell Biol.*, 16 (1963), 187–195.

[32]J. D. Robertson, "The Organization of Cellular Membranes," in *Molecular Organization and Biological Function,* John M. Allen, ed. (New York: Harper & Row, Inc., 1967), 65–106.

[33]T. F. Roth and K. R. Porter, "Specialized Sites on the Cell Surface for Protein Uptake," in *Fifth International Congress for Electron Microscopy*, Philadelphia, Sydney S. Breese Jr., ed., Vol. 2 (New York: Academic Press Inc., 1962), LL-4.

[34]T. F. Roth and K. R. Porter, "Yolk Protein Uptake in the Oocyte of the Mosquito *Aedes aegypti. L.*," *J. Cell Biol.*, 20 (1964), 313–332.

[35]F. S. Sjöstrand, "A New Ultrastructural Element of the Membranes in Mitochondria and of Some Cytoplasmic Membranes," *J. Ultrastruct. Res.*, 9 (1963), 340–361.

[36]F. S. Sjöstrand, "The Structure of Cellular Membranes," *Protoplasma*, 63 (1967), 248–261.

[37]F. S. Sjöstrand, E. A. Cedergren, and U. Karlsson, "Myelin-like Figures Formed from Mitochondrial Material," *Nature*, 202 (1964), 1075–1078.

[38]Donald Svaboda, Harold Grady, and Daniel Azarnoff, "Microbodies in Experimentally Altered Cells," *J. Cell Biol.*, 35 (1967), 127–152.

[39]B. F. Trump and R. E. Bulger, "Studies of Cellular Injury in Isolated Flounder Tubules," *Lab. Invest.*, 16 (1967), 453–482.

[40]D. F. H. Wallach and Adrienne Gordon, "Lipid Protein Interactions in Cellular Membranes," *Fed. Proc.*, 27 (1968), 1263–1268.

[41]M. L. Watson, "Further Observations on the Nuclear Envelope of the Animal Cell," *J. Biophys. Biochem. Cytol.*, 6 (1959), 147–156.

[42]Toshiyuki Yamamoto, "On the Thickness of the Unit Membrane," *J. Cell Biol.*, 17 (1963), 413–421.

IV
STRUCTURAL ENGINEERING IN CELLS

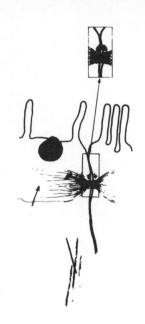

The materials available for construction somewhat limit the type of structure which can be made. When masonry was the main building material, arches were found to be the best means for spanning sizable stretches, and masons fashioned domes from these materials to enclose the tops of buildings. The Industrial Revolution made possible the development of new structural materials with special properties such as cast iron and steel. Since these new materials could serve as a weight-bearing frame, tall buildings such as skyscrapers could be constructed. When the tensile strength of steel was combined and molded with the plastic characteristic of concrete to make reinforced concrete, additional kinds of construction were possible. Throughout history, the true heights of architectual glory have been achieved when harmony was attained between the structural components of a given building and its function.

Structural engineering principles are utilized in cells and in extracellular material. Cells exist in a variety of sizes, shapes, and arrangements, their morphology being related to the type and orientation of the building materials used in their construction. The function of cells is often also related to their form. Some of these basic units of life assume the shape of biconcave discs; others are polyhedral, cuboidal, spherical, flat, or spindle shaped. Nerve and muscle cells are long and may reach many centimeters in length. For example, a single motor neuron may extend from the spinal cord to the toe. On the other hand, the smallest animal cells measure only about 4 microns across. The components found within cells also accomplish specific cell functions. For example, filaments in striated muscle cells enable the cells to contract. Secretory cells often store granules within their cytoplasm which can be released in response to the proper stimulus. This chapter examines some of the components in cells which determine their form and therefore their function.

CELL SHAPE

Molecular Structure and Shape. The shape of some cells appears to be related to their contents. A good example of this relationship is seen in the symmetrical biconcave disc form of the mammalian red blood cell. The red blood cell is small and measures only 4 to 8 microns in diameter. It is filled with hemoglobin molecules that combine with molecular oxygen and carry it to the various tissues of the body. In humans, the red blood cell extrudes its nucleus during development so that the mature cell is enucleate. As the red blood cell develops, it passes through a stage in which it changes from a biconvex to a biconcave form.[25] This change is thought to increase the functional efficiency of the cell. By being disc shaped, rather than spherical, the hemoglobin within the cell can more quickly and completely become saturated with oxygen.[19] The disc shape permits more of the hemoglobin molecules to be closer to the cell surface than would be possible in a spherical cell, where molecules in the center would be some distance away from the surface. The disc shape also permits the cell to change in volume without stretching and rupturing its membrane. Therefore, the biconcave disc shape appears to increase the functional efficiency of the red blood cell. The state of hemoglobin contained within the red cell is fluid enough to permit frequent shape changes. Thus red blood cells can move through passages less than one third of their own diameter without rupturing.[13] This is an advantage to cells that squeeze through small capillaries in the body. It is not known how the mammalian red blood cell accomplishes its change in shape during its development.

Hemoglobin molecules apparently do influence the shape of red blood cells. This is clearly indicated in certain pathological states. For example, *sickle cell anemia* is a hereditary disease in which an abnormal hemoglobin is produced. One of the peptide chains composing the sickle cell hemoglobin molecule has an abnormal sequence of amino acids. A valine residue is substituted for the normal glutamic acid residue. In conditions of low oxygen tension, this defective hemoglobin molecule forms large crystals within the red blood cells. These crystals distort the cell into a sickle shape. Therefore, variations in the molecular structure of sickle cell hemoglobin produce alterations in crystallization that affect the gross shape of red blood cells.

Hereditary spherocytosis is a hematological disease in which red blood cells become spherical and fragile. This disease is associated with a change in the red blood cell membrane, and fragmentation of lipid from it.[22,39] The loss of membrane lipid results in an increased fragility of the red blood cells. The disease is caused by a genetic deletion which alters an enzyme within the membrane of the red cell. Because this enzyme is defective, the cell cannot regulate its volume properly. Therefore, it is unable to extrude, against an external concentration gradient, the excess sodium ions which have diffused into it. As a result, the number of sodium ions continues to increase within the cell, causing an accompanying net influx of water. These two factors cause the cell to swell and become spherical. The cell then becomes changed in shape because its membrane is abnormal.

Attachment Sites. Other structural components also underlie and influence the shape of cells. Attachment sites between adjacent cells are important in this respect. Cells lying free are often spherical, but cells which are bound together to form sheets of tissue have their shapes altered by their relationships with adjacent cells. When the attachment sites between cells are disrupted, the cells change their shapes and frequently round up, taking on the appearance of cells that normally are free of attachments.

A fundamental property of epithelial cells is their tendency to adhere tenaciously to one another along their lateral margins, forming sheets of tissue which line the body cavities and the body surfaces. In electron micrographs, a space measuring approximately 200 Ångström units can be seen between the lateral cell membranes of two adjacent epithelial cells. The exact forces which serve to hold these cells together are unknown but many biologists have suggested the presence of a cementing substance. It is likely that this substance is a mucopolysaccharide. In certain regions the membrane is differentiated into specialized sites of firm cell-to-cell attachment. In epithelial cells, when these specialized contact areas border a free surface or lumen, special types of contact structures have been identified and collectively are referred to as a *junctional complex*.[10] Junctional complex areas (Fig. IV–1) consist of three separate elements: (1) a *tight junction,* (2) an *intermediate junction,* and (3) a *desmosome*. However, more recent studies indicate that another highly specialized area of contact, known as a *gap junction,* also exists in isolated regions between epithelial cells.[31] The structure of gap junctions is considered later in this chapter.

The tight junction borders the luminal surface of the epithelial cells (Fig. III–2). It is formed when the external leaflets of the lateral unit membranes of two adjoining cells fuse. In certain epithelia, the fusion of the membranes appears to obliterate the intercellular space in the area of contact, thus forming a barrier to the penetration of large molecules.

This tight junction region can be visualized as a zone encircling the entire luminal perimeter of the cell. It therefore acts as an effective seal to prevent the passage of tracer substances from the lumen into the intercellular spaces.

More recent studies indicate that there are different kinds of tight junctions. In many capillaries the tight junctions which exist between neighboring endothelial cells are only spots of membrane fusion, rather than being continuous thick belts extending around the luminal perimeter of the cells. This was discovered in studies using the small protein tracer horseradish peroxidase.[23] In electron micrographs, peroxidase particles (having a radius of about 25 Ångström units) were found localized in the intercellular clefts between adjacent capillary endothelial cells. This was taken as evidence that the endothelial cell-to-cell junctions were permeable to the small tracer. A 40-Ångström-unit space was detected between adjacent endothelial cell membranes in areas previously thought to be tight junctions. Because these junctions allowed the passage of horseradish peroxidase,[23] they could not be considered functionally as true tight junctions. Apparently, small molecules and ions are able to pass through these junctions, indicating that they could serve as an important route for the diffusion of certain substances. Notable exceptions, however, are found in capillaries of the lung, retina, and brain, where true tight junctions (fused zones encircling the entire perimeter of the cells) exist.[30] These tight junctions *prevent* the intercellular passage of peroxidase and other large substances from the blood into the tissue.

Recently, another highly specialized junction has been described. In certain electrical synapses it was reported that the membrane surfaces of the adjacent nerve cells were characterized by hexagonally packed subunits.[32] Similar hexagonal arrangements were also reported in isolated liver plasma membranes.[3] It has now been discovered, primarily through the use of the electron-opaque substance lanthanum, that certain cell junctions in a number of different tissues display a characteristic hexagonal pattern (Fig. IV–2).[31] Lanthanum is able to enter spaces in these junctions (for this reason they have been called gap junctions) and thus outline the hexagonal pattern which exists on the apposing junctional cell membranes. *En face* views of gap junction membranes subjected to the lanthanum technique clearly display a highly structured hexagonal pattern. Studies employing freeze-etching also support the finding that hexagonal subunits comprise gap junction membranes. Models have been proposed to correlate the structure of gap junctions with the low electrical resistance presumably located here,[27] but more information is necessary before we fully understand the significance of these contact areas between cells.

Many adjacent epithelial cells have both tight junctions (which exist as part of the junctional complex) and isolated gap junctional regions. The tight junction prevents the flow of large molecules into the intercellular space between the cells, and compartmentalizes the basal and apical environments of the epithelium (defining an "inside" and "outside" surface). The gap junction appears to couple the epithelium into a functional unity, by creating a low resistance pathway between the cytoplasm of adjacent epithelial cells.

Although we have been discussing junctions in epithelia, it is worth noting here that between smooth muscle cells localized regions of contact also occur. The outer leaflets of the unit membranes surrounding adjacent cells appear to form gap junctions, similar in structure to those just discussed. This form of contact between adjacent smooth muscle cells has been termed a *nexus*. [8,9] The word nexus means a bond between members of a group and suggests that this junction permits a special form of communication between these cells. The nexus has a low electrical resistance and therefore appears to permit the passage of ions from cell to cell. This allows excitation to spread easily throughout the smooth muscle tissue. It therefore appears that the nexus and the gap junction are similar (if not identical) regions of contact between cells.

Another part of the junctional complex is the intermediate junction (Fig. IV–1). It exists adjacent and basal to the tight junction and encircles the cell as a belt-like zone. An intercellular space, containing moderately dense material and measuring approximately 200 Ångström units across, separates the adjacent cell membranes in this region. The adjacent cytoplasm of the cells contains dense filamentous material. This material presumably contributes structural stability to the intermediate junction. The function of the intermediate junction is unknown.

The desmosome (Fig. IV–1) is an additional element of the junctional complex. This structure is a spot-like specialization formed by dense cytoplasmic plaques lying parallel to the inner leaflet of each cell membrane. An intercellular space, about 250 Ångström units wide, separates the two halves of the desmosome. This space contains a central layer of dense material. Cytoplasmic filaments are associated with the desmosomal plaques. Sometimes the filaments loop into the area of the plaque [24] or sometimes they run parallel with it (Fig. IV–3). Desmosomes are not immediately continuous with the intermediate junction of the junctional complex but are usually located some distance from it. Isolated desmosomes are also found along the lateral borders of epithelial cells as well. Desmosomes are thought to be spots of permanent structural contact between cells. When tissue shrinks, the cells often remain attached by the desmosome region. In earlier times, these desmosome-linked extensions were thought to be points of true cytoplasmic interconnection—actual bridges—between cells. This is not after all the case, since an intercellular space is always present in these areas.

Heart muscle displays a number of cell junctions called *intercalated discs* by the light microscopists. These junctions, which exist at the ends of cardiac muscle cells, appear as dark bands in electron micrographs and are composed of all elements of the junctional complex (Fig. IV–4). However, in heart muscle the membrane modifications do not exhibit the precise topographical relationship often found in epithelia.

Intercalated discs display a complex structure.[5,11] Cytoplasmic processes from adjacent cardiac cells interdigitate to form an interlocking relationship between the ends of the cells. Interspersed along this undulating contour are desmosomes, intermediate junctions, and spot-like tight junctions. Myofilaments from the cells converge upon the intermediate junctions and desmosomes. In addition to the tight junctional sites which exist along the intercalated discs, there are large areas along the longitudinal cell boundaries where the membranes appear to form gap junctions.[31] These extensive gap junctional areas create low-resistance electrical pathways, so that excitation can easily spread throughout the entire heart muscle.[11] This is similar to the specialized nexus junction that exists in smooth muscle.

In many invertebrate epithelia, tight junctions and gap junctions are replaced by a *septate junction,* which may perform the function both of insulation and coupling. In these junctions the normal intercellular space does not become smaller but instead is occluded for several microns by a series of septa, spaced at regular intervals. In face view, these junctions appear to be composed of hexagonal subunits. Some studies have shown gap junctions to exist in these tissues as well as septate junctions. Molecules of several thousand molecular weight have been shown to pass from one cell cytoplasm to the next (presumably via one of these two types of junctions) without entering the extracellular fluid.[26,40]

Calcium Ions and Cell Association. The ionic environment of a cell profoundly affects its shape. For some time it has been recognized that calcium ions are important in maintaining cell adhesiveness. Tissues placed in calcium-free media soon reveal separations between their cells, and elements of the junctional complexes disappear.[6,20,28,35] The role that calcium ions play in maintaining cell cohesiveness is not understood, but removal of this ion causes striking alterations in cell architecture. As various parts of the junctional complex are disrupted (by a lack of calcium), the cells show drastic morphological changes (Fig. IV–5).[6] Their normal orientation is lost and they detach from their neighbors (Fig. IV–6). Becoming free, they assume a spherical shape. In these cases the desmosomes separate and strands of material are left bridging the gap between the apposing cell membranes.

The importance of calcium ion in permitting dissociated cells to reassociate has been demonstrated in experiments with sponges.[21] Following certain experimental treatments sponge cells can be separated from each other. Only when sufficient calcium ions are present will the sponge cells reassociate. Therefore, the presence of calcium ion in the medium is essential for cell reassociation and for the differentiation and maintenance of cell junctions.

Filaments. Filaments also contribute to the structural framework of cells. Feltworks of extremely fine filaments have been seen in the apical regions of epithelial cells and forming a core in the finger-like processes of cells called *microvilli* (Fig. IV–7). Additional filaments and/or amorphous material run parallel to the cell surface forming what has been called a *terminal web.** Other larger filaments (sometimes called tonofilaments) course throughout the cytoplasm of cells, presumably helping to maintain cell shape. These filaments diverge into the region of the desmosome.

If junctional complex attachment sites are experimentally altered so that the cells come apart, cytoplasmic filaments are still evident, but the cells change their shape.[6] The filaments therefore appear to act as guy wires, providing tensile strength. In addition, filaments associated with the special areas of cell attachment appear to provide a supportive framework.

Microtubules and the Maintenance of Cell Form. Microtubules are long thin cylindrical inclusions that exist in plant and animal cells (Fig. IV–8). They are straight or gently curving uniform structures several microns long and measuring 200 to 270 Ångström units in diameter.[11] Their center displays a low electron density, which makes them appear hollow (Fig. IV–9). The wall of each microtubule has been reported to consist of thirteen subfilaments. The distribution of microtubules within various cells has offered clues as to their function in the formation and maintenance of cell shape. Perhaps the best evidence for the function of microtubules comes from studies of certain protozoa. *Tokophrya* is one such organism that has many long (30 to 50 microns), slender (1 micron in diameter) tentacles extending from the periphery of the cell.[33] These tentacles are remarkably straight, rigid, protoplasmic extensions that are used to capture food. The top of the tentacle appears to bore a hole through the body wall of the prey and remain attached to it; then, during the feeding process, cytoplasm from the prey flows down the center portion of the tentacle into food vacuoles within the *Tokophrya*. At the same time, smaller granules thought to contain digestive enzymes or toxic chemicals which serve to immobilize the prey can be observed moving in the opposite direction in a more peripheral channel within the tentacle. Electron microscopical observations of a cross section of a tentacle reveals a patterned array of microtubules within this protoplasmic extension. The arrangement of the microtubules creates two distinct passageways; a large, central one about 300 microns in diameter permits food to flow into *Tokophrya*. Peripheral to the outer set of microtubules, within the confines of the plasma membrane, is a narrow channel where granules

---

*More than one type of intracellular filament can be found. Fine filaments 50 to 70 Ångström units identified in some cells may be formed from actin-like proteins and be involved in cell movement or contraction.

may pass to the prey. It appears that microtubules in *Tokophrya* not only function to maintain tentacle shape, but they also guide the streaming of particles and may in some unexplained way also provide the motive force.

Microtubules (called neurotubules) are also seen in the long processes of nerve cells. Substances from nerve cell bodies have been observed to move to the ends of these long cytoplasmic processes. Therefore, by analogy to *Tokophrya* it appears that microtubules may also be related to the shape of nerve cell processes and to the movement of materials (originating at the cell body) along them.

Microtubules also appear to play a role in pigment cells. Melanophores are cells abundant in fish skin which contain a large number of melanin pigment granules. Movement of the pigment granules into the cytoplasmic processes (expansion) is associated with darkening of the fish, while blanching occurs when the melanin pigment moves into the cell body (contraction). It has been discovered that the pigment granules are arranged in rows or channels which are delimited by microtubules.[4,37] Apparently the microtubules act as guides or tracts for the movement of the pigment granules.[29,17]

An obvious role for microtubules is the maintenance of cell form. As discussed previously, it appears that they are the elements supporting the long, slender, rigid tentacles in *Tokophrya*. Additional evidence for a cytoskeletal function of microtubules comes from studies on the multinucleated protozoan *Actinosphaerium (Echinosphaerium)*.[37] This unusual organism has very long, slender protoplasmic processes called axopods extending peripherally from it in all directions. These axopods are used for locomotion and feeding. They measure 400 to 500 microns in length and are about 10 to 15 microns in diameter at their bases. The core of each axopod consists of an interlocking double-coiled array of microtubules which appear to be responsible for the shape and support of the process. Exposing *Actinosphaerium* to low temperature and/or high pressure causes the axopods to form nubbin-like processes which soon withdraw into the body. These supporting structures gradually disappear or solate. Electron microscopical examination of the nubbin structures show that their microtubules have disassembled, presumably by depolymerization, into a finely amorphous material. The axopods can be made to reappear if treated *Actinosphaerium* specimens are returned to higher temperatures and normal pressures. Ultrastructural examination of reformed axopods reveals the presence of microtubules which presumably have repolymerized from the amorphous filamentous material. These and other studies suggest that cytoplasmic gel formation (resulting in a rigid protoplasmic structure) is probably associated with polymerization of proteins that results in the formation of microtubules.[29]

Microtubules also appear to be related to cell form in nucleated blood cells. A densely staining band of material was seen to rim fish red blood cells and appeared to be related to the maintenance of their shape. It was shown that this band was formed by a group of microtubules.[12]

Blood platelets also have a marginal bundle of microtubules that appear to be responsible for their lenticular shape. Platelets exposed to the cold become spherical; at the same time the marginal bundle disappears.[2] Rewarming platelets to body temperature for 1 hour causes the bundle of microtubules to reform and the lentiform shape of the platelet returns. Occasionally, rewarmed platelets assume cigar shapes. When these cigar-shaped platelets are examined electron microscopically, their microtubules are seen to be arranged in a central, straight bundle that lies parallel to the long axis.

It should be clear from the foregoing that no single mechanism or structure is responsible for overall determination of cell shape. Only the complex interaction of structures such as microtubules, filaments, desmosomes, and so forth, formed and genetically determined in a given cell milieu, really determines precise form.

CELL MOVEMENT

Cells undergo different kinds of movement, which are in part dependent upon the same sorts of arrangement that determine their shape. In fact, some cell movements are simply directed changes in shape. For example, white blood cells and amoebae undergo a form of locomotion, called amoeboid movement, whereby they displace themselves from one site to another. In this process they manifest obvious external deformations. Some cells have restricted their shape changes to appendages which move. Cilia and flagella are examples of such cell appendages capable of active movement. If the ciliated cells are attached into a layer, the beating of the cilia can serve to propel material along their surfaces. If the cells are free and have a single or multiple cilia or flagella, the cell can be propelled, as in the case of sperm cells. These primitive types of movement are characteristic of eucaryotic cells of many phyla and are discussed briefly below. Muscle cells bring about another kind of movement. The filaments present within muscle cells cause the cells to shorten. Because these cells are attached to the skeleton, the shortening brings about gross movement. Muscle contraction is one of the best studied examples of the relations of macromolecular structure to cell function. This is examined in some detail in Chapter VII.

AMOEBOID MOVEMENT

Although most cells are more or less fixed in shape, amoebae have a shape that is variable. An amoeba actively changes shape as it sends forth cytoplasmic projections called *pseudopods*. The pseudopods are responsible for the direction of movement. As protoplasm from the main

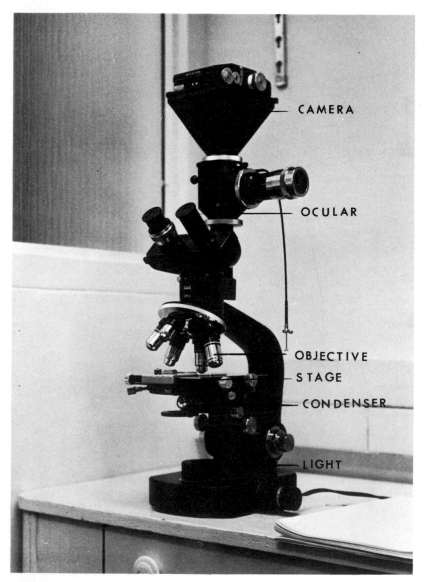

CAMERA

OCULAR

OBJECTIVE

STAGE

CONDENSER

LIGHT

FIGURE I–1. A type of light microscope commonly used in biological research. Photograph by Miss Leslie Caldwell.

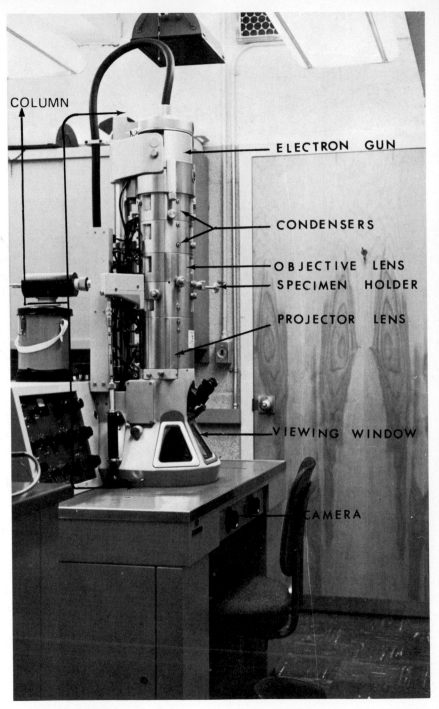

COLUMN

ELECTRON GUN

CONDENSERS

OBJECTIVE LENS
SPECIMEN HOLDER
PROJECTOR LENS

VIEWING WINDOW

CAMERA

FIGURE I–2. An electron microscope ready for use in a research laboratory. Photograph by Miss Leslie Caldwell.

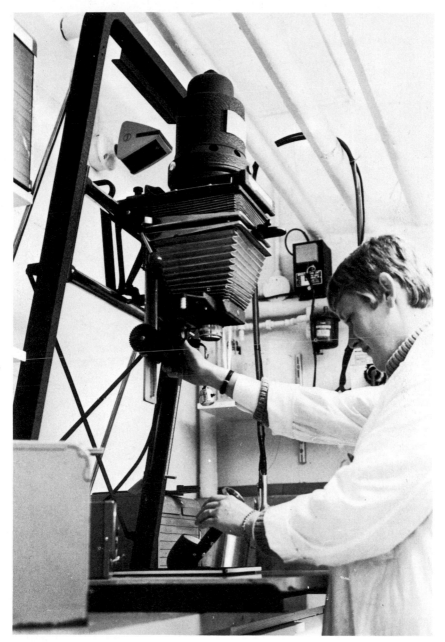

FIGURE I–3. Enlarging. Negatives taken with a light or electron microscope are magnified in this enlarger and printed to produce permanent records of the material.

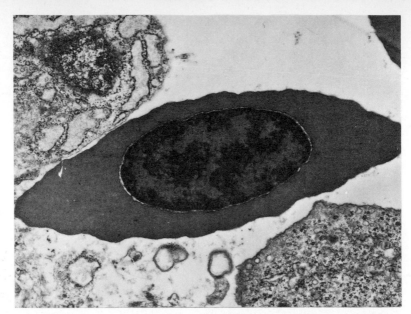

FIGURE I–4. Electron micrograph of a nucleated fish erythrocyte as seen after chemical fixation and thin sectioning (so-called "conventional techniques"). The cytoplasm of this cell is relatively homogeneous and uncomplicated by organelles. The large, ovoid nucleus has many nuclear pores in its surrounding membrane which are difficult to detect in such preparations. × 14,900. Micrograph courtesy of Dr. J. K. Koehler.

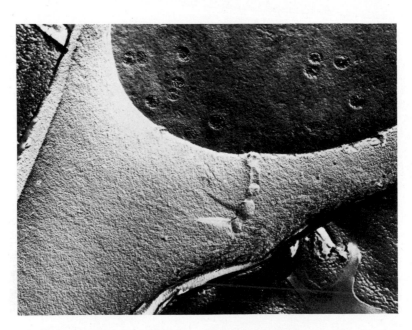

FIGURE I–5. Electron micrograph of a portion of a nucleated frog erythrocyte examined by means of the freeze-etching technique. This method creates a three-dimensional replica of the cell, which allows various surfaces to be visualized. Note that the round nuclear pores now are quite obvious structures. × 23,500. Micrograph courtesy of Dr. J. K. Koehler.

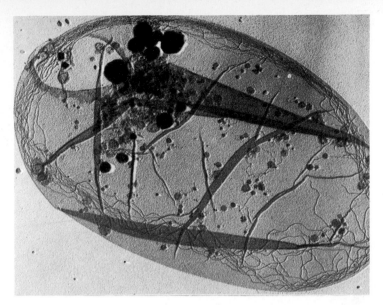

FIGURE I–6. Electron micrograph of a nucleated frog erythrocyte (ghost) which has been lysed is shown here in a shadowed preparation. The hole in the erythrocyte membrane at the upper left presumably represents the site of lysis. The bulk of the cytoplasm and nucleus are absent, leaving only a few dense mitochondria, some small vesicular organelles, and the prominent "marginal band" of microtubules, which give this cell support. × 5,700. Micrograph courtesy of Dr. J. K. Koehler.

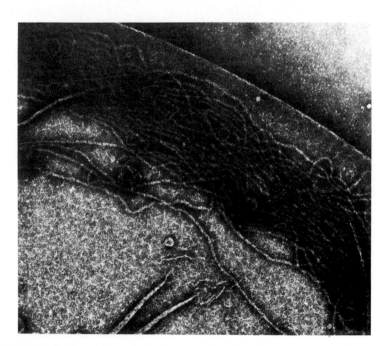

FIGURE I–7. Electron micrograph of a small region of the periphery of a nucleated frog erythrocyte (ghost) is seen via the method of negative staining in this figure. × 19,900. Micrograph courtesy of Dr. J. K. Koehler.

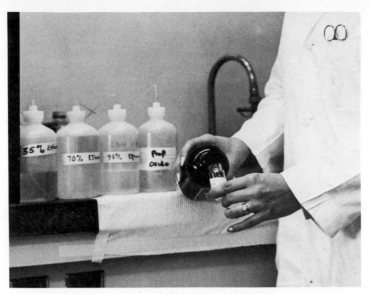

FIGURE I–8. Dehydration. After the tissue is fixed, the water is removed by placing the tissue in a series of alcohols of increasing concentration before it is embedded. Photograph by Miss Leslie Caldwell.

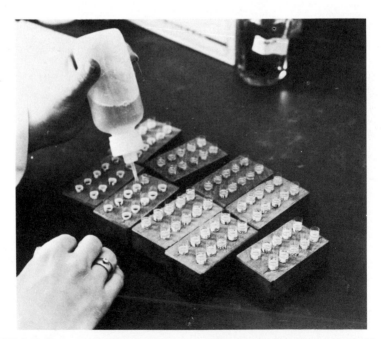

FIGURE I–9. Embedding. Small geletin capsules are filled with liquid plastic resin and then the tissue is placed on the surface of the plastic. The tissue sinks. The plastic is subsequently hardened forming a block containing the tissue. Photograph by Joseph Ewing.

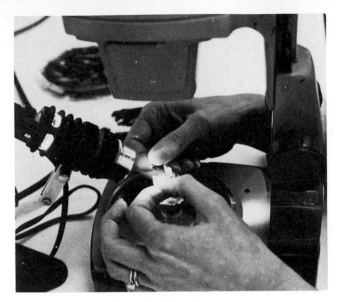

FIGURE I–10. **T**rimming. The excess plastic is trimmed from the hardened block prior to sectioning. Photograph by Joseph Ewing.

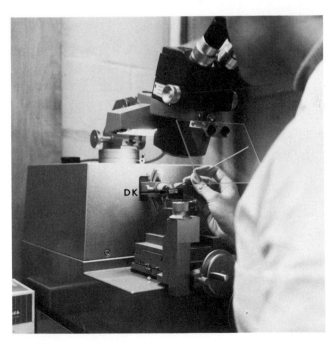

FIGURE I–11. **T**hin sectioning. The trimmed plastic *block* is placed in an ultramicrotome and sectioned using *glass or diamond knives* (DK). Sections float onto the surface of the water in a boat containing the knife, and the grids are picked up for viewing in the electron microscope. Photograph by Miss Leslie Caldwell.

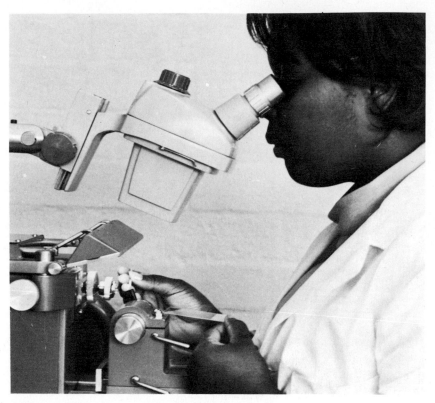

FIGURE I–12. Thick sectioning. Thicker sections can be cut from the plastic block, mounted on glass slides, and viewed in a light microscope. Photograph by Joseph Ewing.

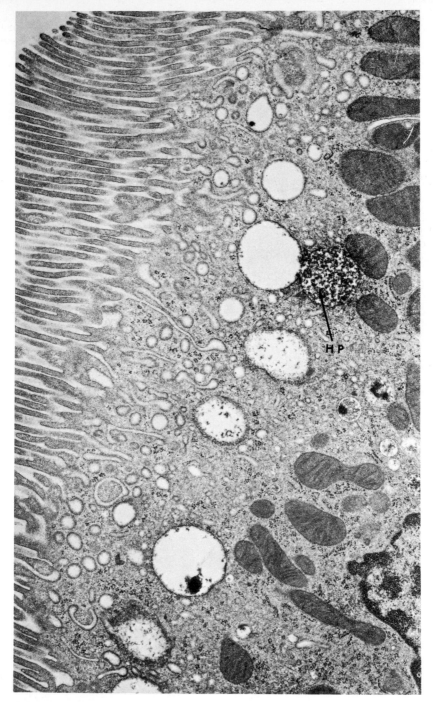

FIGURE I–13. Electron micrograph of a proximal convoluted tubular cell from the nephron showing the tracer horseradish peroxidase (HP) within apical vacuoles. × 12,800.

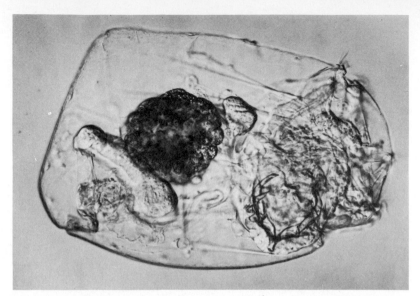

FIGURE I–14. The rotifer (wheel animalcule) *Asplanchna sieboldi* in the living state as seen in the Nomarski interference microscope. The jaws are seen embedded in the muscular "pharynx" at the lower right. × 160. Micrograph courtesy of Dr. John Gilbert, Dartmouth College. From the article by J. K. Koehler and T. L. Hayes, *J. Ultrastruct. Res.* 27 (1969), 419.

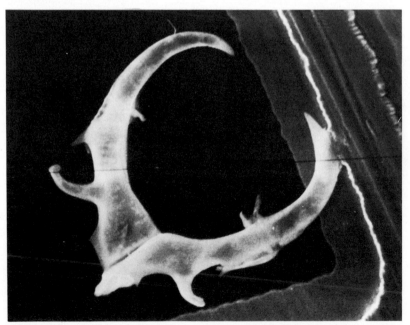

FIGURE I–15. Isolated jaws of the rotifer *Asplanchna* as seen in the scanning electron microscope. The various projections and appendages of the jaws are more easily recognized in such preparations. × 2,400. Micrograph courtesy of J. K. Koehler and T. L. Hayes, *J. Ultrastruct. Res.* 27 (1969), 419.

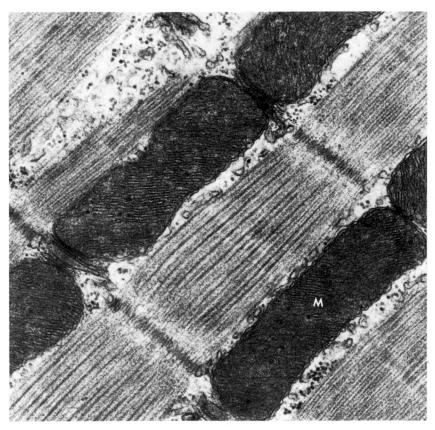

FIGURE II–5. Electron micrograph showing the alignment of the myofilaments. Note the close association of these filaments with mitochondria (M). × 33,300.

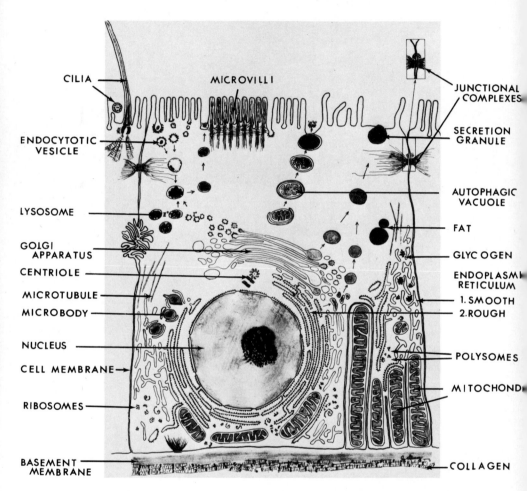

FIGURE III–1. Schematic diagram of a cell showing the major organelles.

CILIA

MICROVILLI

JUNCTIONAL COMPLEXES

ENDOCYTOTIC VESICLE

SECRETION GRANULE

AUTOPHAGIC VACUOLE

LYSOSOME

FAT

GOLGI APPARATUS

GLYCOGEN

CENTRIOLE

ENDOPLASMIC RETICULUM

MICROTUBULE

1. SMOOTH

MICROBODY

2. ROUGH

NUCLEUS

POLYSOMES

CELL MEMBRANE

RIBOSOMES

MITOCHONDRIA

BASEMENT MEMBRANE

COLLAGEN

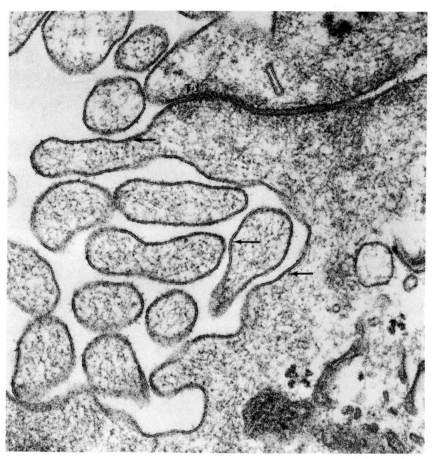

FIGURE III–2. Electron micrograph showing the unit membrane structure (arrow) of an apical cell membrane. At the lateral borders of two adjacent cells, the outer leaflets of the unit membranes fuse, forming a tight junction (TJ) region. × 75,900.

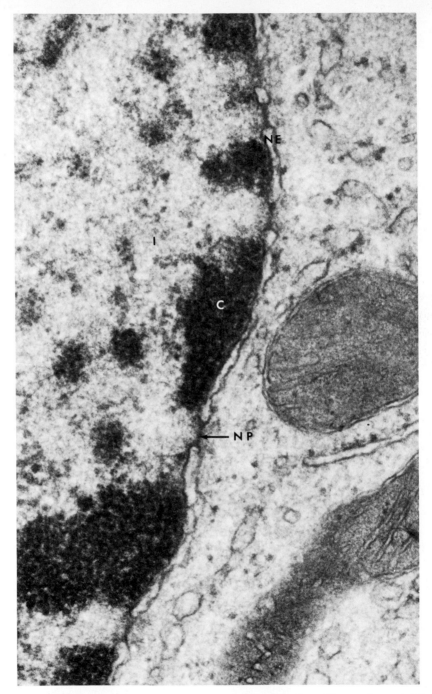

FIGURE III–3. Electron micrograph showing part of a nucleus. The nucleus contains chromatin material (C) and interchromatin (I) material. The nucleoplasm is separated from the cytoplasm by a double-walled sac, the nuclear envelope (NE). The sac is interrupted periodically by nuclear pores (NP). × 79,800.

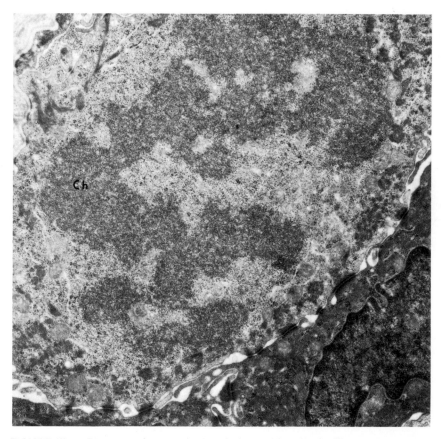

FIGURE III–4. Electron micrograph showing a cell in mitosis. The nuclear envelope has disappeared and the chromatin material is condensed to form chromosomes (Ch). × 11,300.

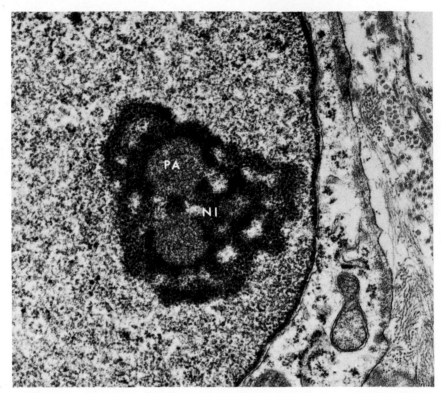

FIGURE III–5. Electron micrograph showing part of a nucleus containing a nucleolus. The nucleolus is formed of a nucleolonema (NI) and a pars amorpha (PA). Note granular composition of the peripheral area of the nucleolonema. The granules are ribosomal precursors. × 28,000.

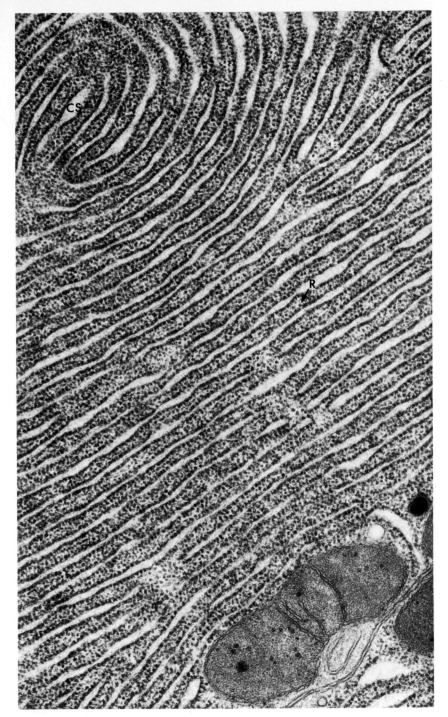

FIGURE III–6. Electron micrograph showing an oriented array of parallel cisternae of rough-surfaced endoplasmic reticulum from a protein secreting cell of the exocrine pancreas. Ribosome (R); cisternal space (CS). × 33,000.

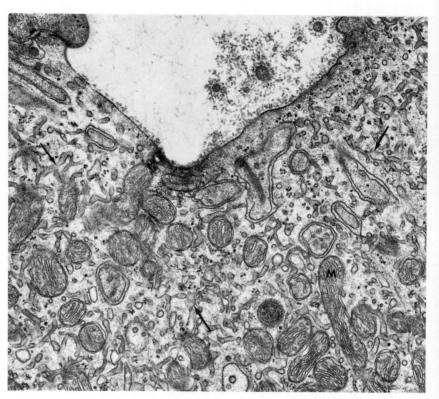

FIGURE III–7. Electron micrograph showing smooth-surfaced endoplasmic reticulum (arrows) in a chloride-secreting cell from a fish gill. Mitochondria are also abundant in this cell type. × 20,100.

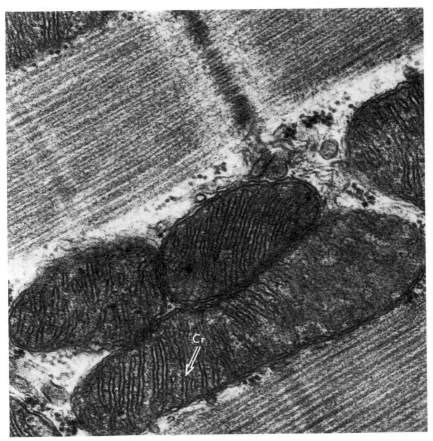

FIGURE III–8. Electron micrograph showing several mitochondria in the cytoplasm of a striated muscle cell. Cristae (Cr). × 52,700.

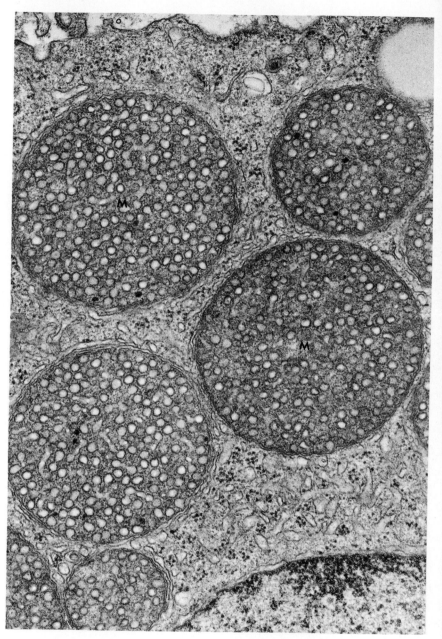

FIGURE III–9. Electron micrograph showing mitochondria (M) in the cytoplasm of a cell from the adrenal cortex. In this case the cristae of the mitochondria appear to be tubular. × 40,200. Micrograph courtesy of Dr. Daniel Friend.

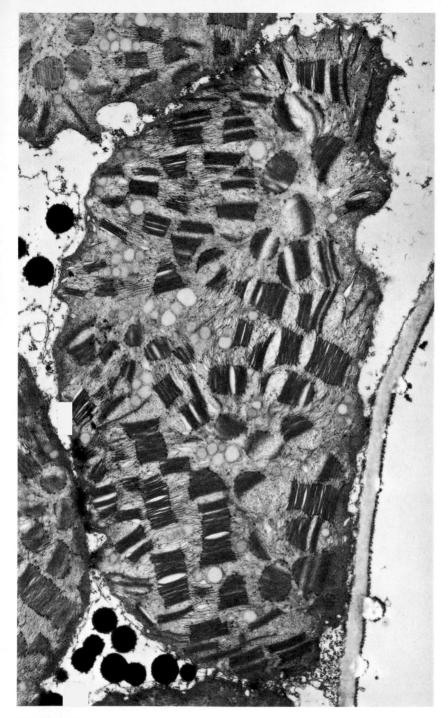

FIGURE III–10. Electron micrograph showing a chloroplast from an African violet plant. × 17,300. Micrograph courtesy of Mrs. Carlotta M. Roach.

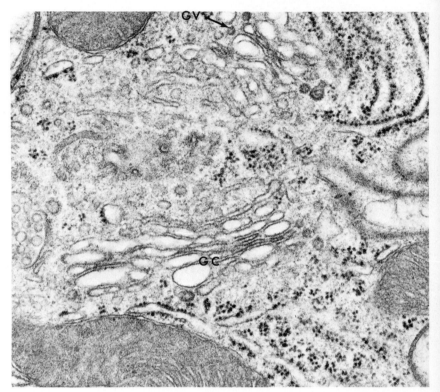

FIGURE III–11. Electron micrograph showing a Golgi area in a kidney cell. Stacks of closely spaced Golgi cisternae (GC) are surrounded by a few Golgi vesicles (GV). × 32,700.

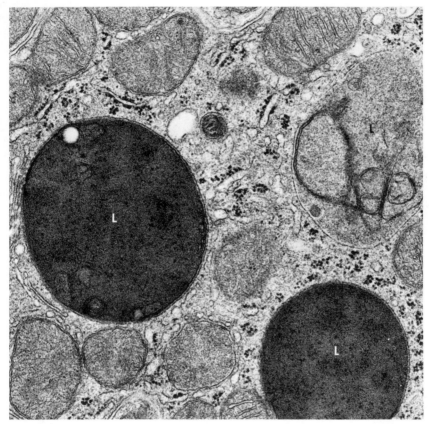

FIGURE III–12. Electron micrograph showing three lysosomes (L). Two of them have an electron-dense matrix and one has an electron-lucent matrix. All three contain additional material. × 31,800.

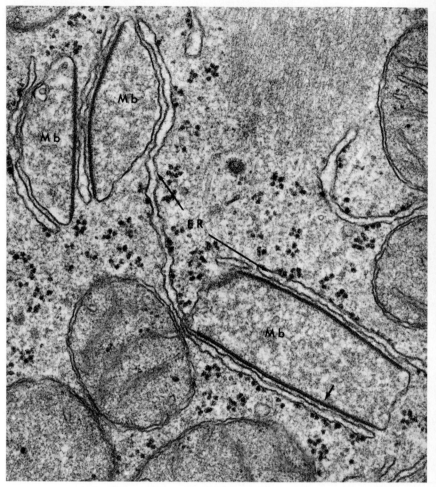

FIGURE III–13. Electron micrograph showing several microbodies (Mb) (peroxisomes) from a kidney proximal tubular cell. × 50,300.

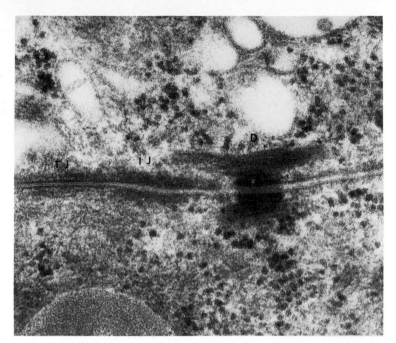

FIGURE IV–1. Electron micrograph showing the three elements which comprise a junctional complex. They are found at the luminal surface and consist of the tight junction (TJ); the intermediate junction (IJ); and the desmosome (D). × 62,600.

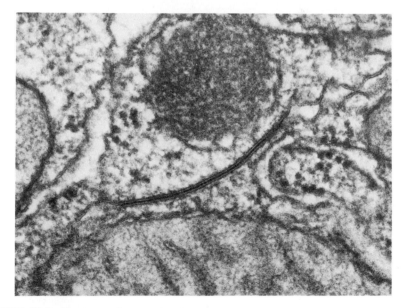

FIGURE IV–2. Electron micrograph of a gap junction from kidney tissue. The gap is infiltrated with colloidal lanthanum. × 84,600. Micrograph courtesy of Dr. Fred Silver-blatt.

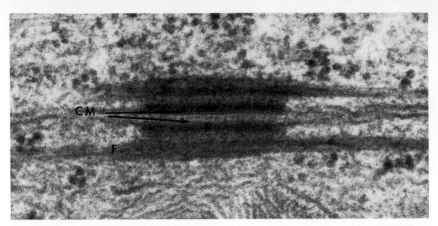

FIGURE IV–3. Electron micrograph showing a desmosome. Filaments (F) can be seen running through the cytoplasm adjacent to, and associated with, the desmosome. A dense plaque (P) lies underneath the unit membrane of each cell. Dense material can be seen between the two cell membranes (CM) in the intercellular space. × 86,100.

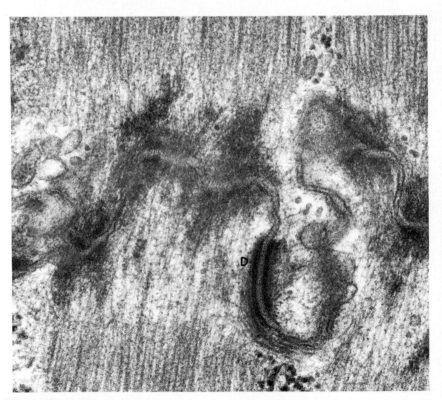

FIGURE IV–4. Electron micrograph showing an intercalated disc from cardiac muscle. Some areas of the cell membranes are obliquely sectioned and therefore appear as areas of gray density. Desmosomes (D), tight junction regions, and intermediate junction regions can be found along the course of such discs. × 55,300.

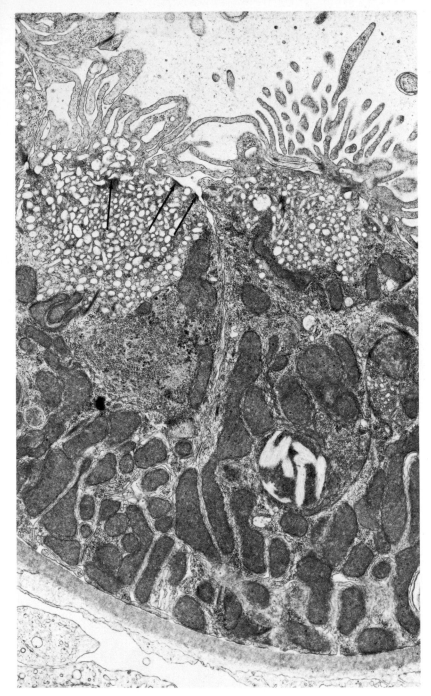

FIGURE IV–5. Electron micrograph showing cells from a flounder kidney tubule which was incubated in a medium free of calcium ions. The junctional complexes (arrows) are coming apart and disappearing. × 10,200. From the article by R. E. Bulger and B. F. Trump, *J. Ultrastruct Res.* 28 (1969), 301.

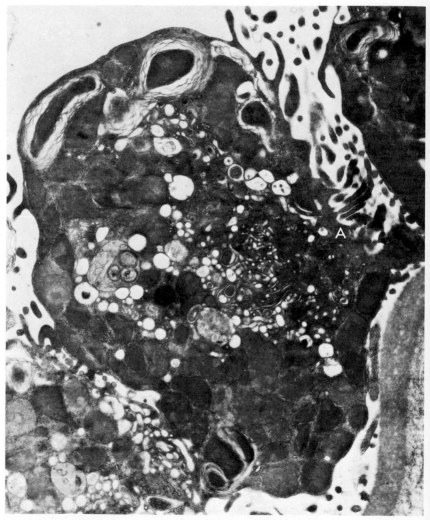

FIGURE IV–6. Electron micrograph taken of a flounder kidney tubule which was incubated in a medium lacking calcium ions. At this time period, the kidney cells have become completely separated from their neighbors and in fact have turned around within the basement membrane so that the apical (A) region of the cell is now extending laterally. × 5,000.

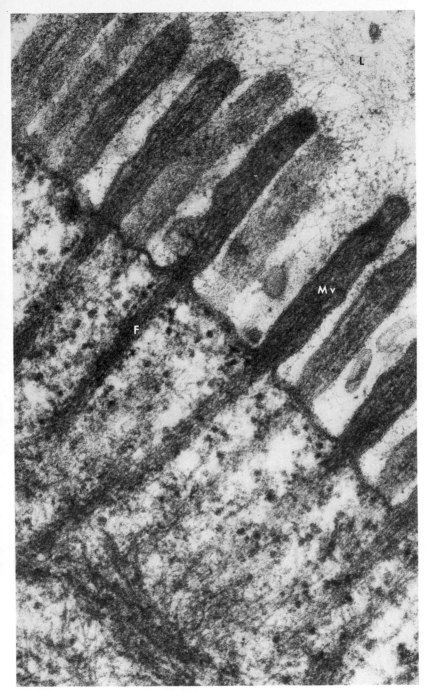

FIGURE IV–7. Electron micrograph showing the apical region of a columnar absorptive cell from the small intestine. Microvilli (Mv) extend into the lumen (L). Within the microvilli are bundles of filaments (F), which extend down into the cytoplasm below. × 73,300.

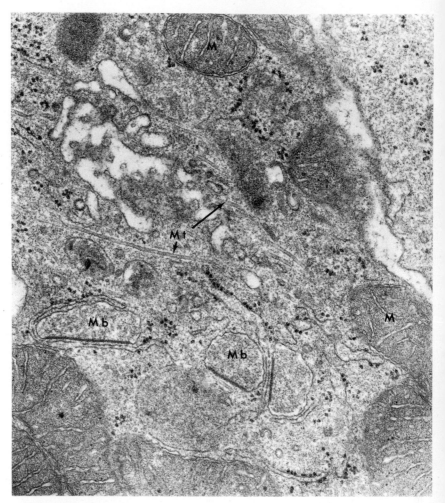

FIGURE IV–8. Electron micrograph showing microtubules (arrow) running through the cytoplasm between mitochondria (M) and microbodies (Mb). × 33,500.

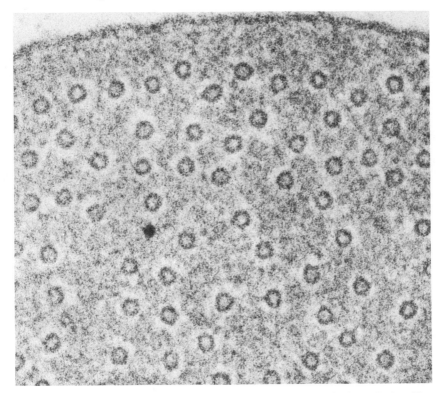

FIGURE IV–9. Electron micrograph showing cross sections of microtubules. These microtubules are approximately 250 Angstrom units in diameter and have a pale staining core which makes them appear hollow. They are surrounded by an electron-lucent area of cytoplasm forming a halo. × 175,200.

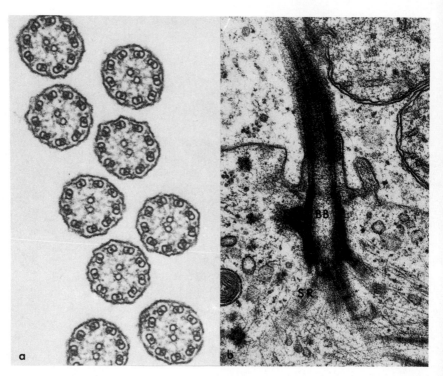

FIGURE IV–10a. Electron micrograph showing a cross section of several cilia and the 9 + 2 pattern. The nine peripheral doublets and two single central units are microtubules. An extension of the cell membrane surrounds the cilia. × 57,700.

FIGURE IV–10b. Electron micrograph showing a cilium protruding from the apex of the cell. It is anchored in a basal body (BB) or modified centriole by striated rootlet (SR) fibers. × 40,000.

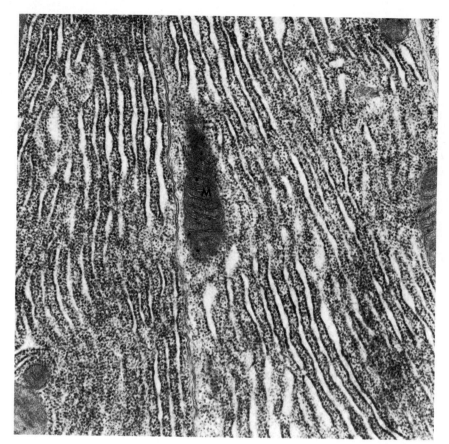

FIGURE V–8. Electron micrograph showing a portion of cytoplasm from an exocrine pancreas cell filled with rough-surfaced endoplasmic reticulum. The small black dots represent ribosomes which are lined up along the surface of the membrane sacs. The protein is produced on the ribosome and transferred into the lumen of the membrane sacs. A few mitochondria (M) are also present in the micrograph. × 22,600.

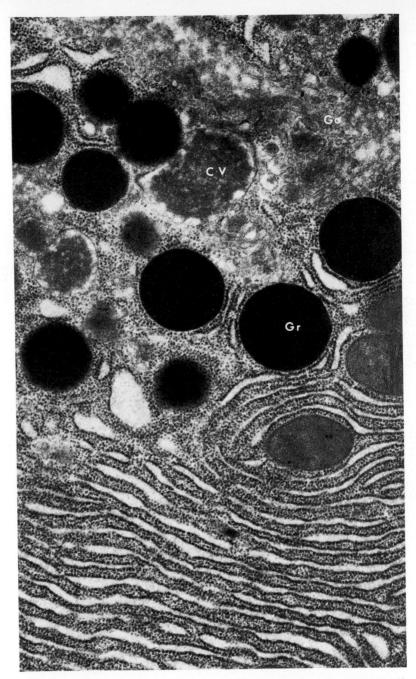

FIGURE V–9. Electron micrograph showing the rough-surfaced endoplasmic reticulum at the bottom of the picture. The protein moves within the cisternae of the endoplasmic reticulum into the Golgi zone (Go) where it is condensed in condensing vacuoles (CV). The condensed secretory product is stored in the cytoplasm of the cells as dense granules (Gr). × 24,300.

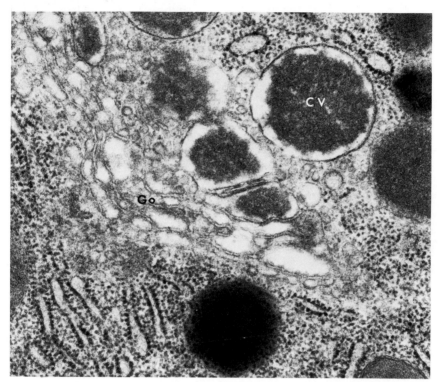

FIGURE V–10. Electron micrograph showing another Golgi region (Go) from an exocrine pancreas cell. The secretory product is condensed within the condensing vacuole (CV). × 39,500.

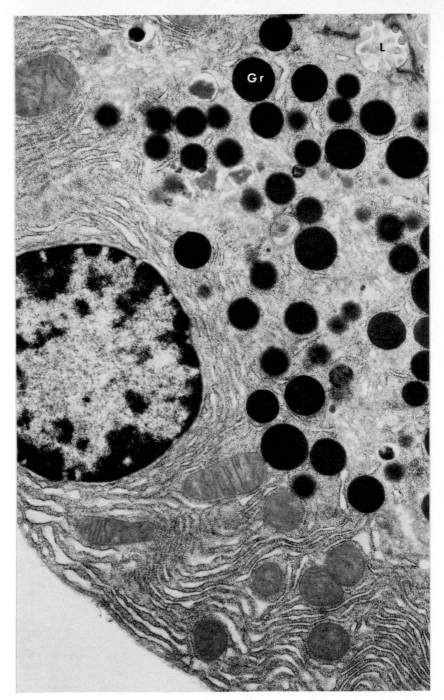

FIGURE V–11. Electron micrograph of an exocrine pancreas cell showing the stored secretory granules (Gr) in the apex of the cell. A small lumen (L) is seen in the upper right. × 12,600.

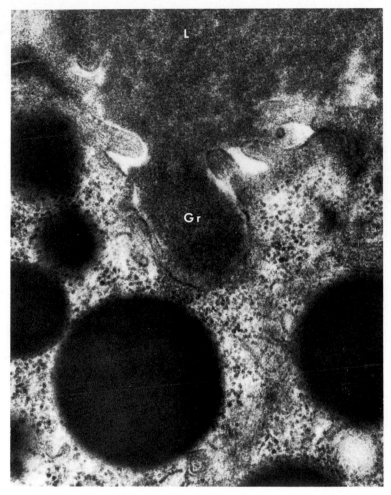

FIGURE V–12. Electron micrograph showing the release of a secreted granule (Gr) into the lumen (L). × 43,900.

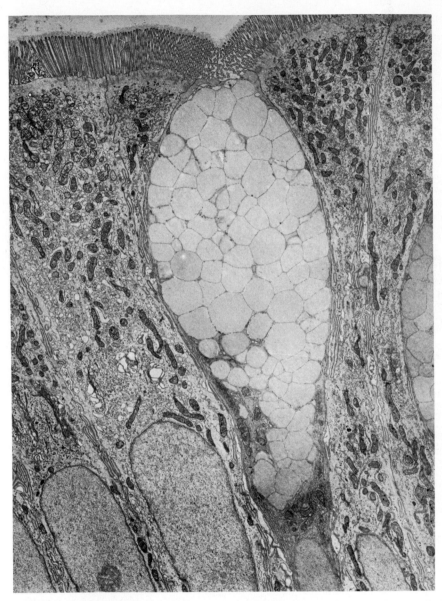

FIGURE V–13. Electron micrograph showing parts of two goblet cells in the intestine. The basal region of the cell contains a nucleus and some rough-surfaced endoplasmic reticulum. The remaining cytoplasm is filled with mucous granules. × 7,100. Electron micrograph courtesy of Dr. Guido Tytgat.

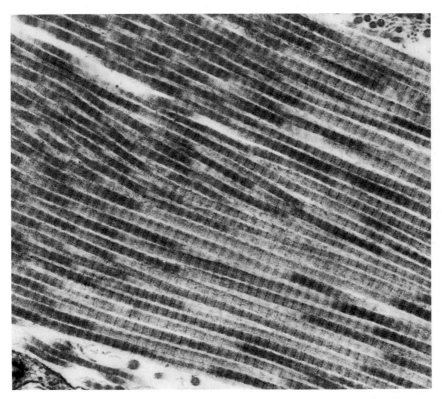

FIGURE V–14. Electron micrograph showing extracellular bundles of collagen fibrils. The fibrils have a characteristic 700-Ångström-unit cross striation. × 36,600.

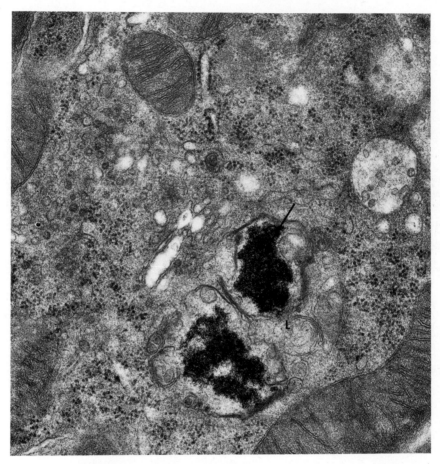

FIGURE VI–1. Electron micrograph showing a lysosome (L) from a kidney tubular cell. The tissue has been reacted to demonstrate acid phosphatase activity, which can be seen as black reaction product (arrow) within the lysosome. × 29,900.

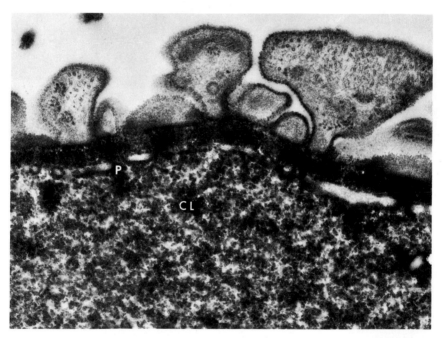

FIGURE VI–2. Electron micrograph showing the protein horseradish peroxidase being filtered from the capillary lumen (CL) through the endothelial pores (P) and through the substance of the basement membrane of a renal corpuscle. × 24,900.

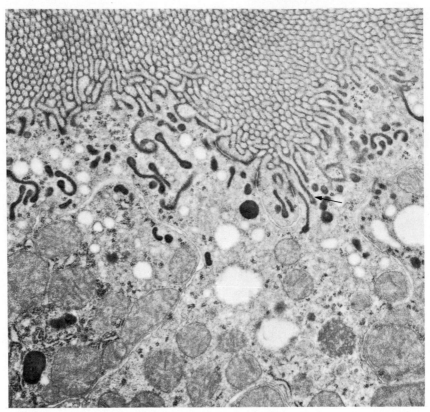

FIGURE VI–3. Electron micrograph showing the dense reaction product of the horseradish peroxidase within the apical tubular invaginations (arrow) in the apical region of the proximal convoluted tubular cells from a nephron. × 11,200.

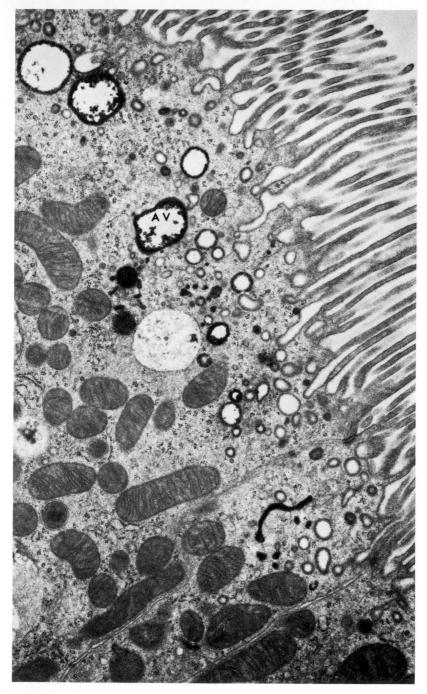

FIGURE VI–4. Electron micrograph showing the dense reaction product formed at the site of the enzyme horseradish peroxidase within the vesicles of the apical cytoplasm and within larger apical vacuoles (AV). × 12,500.

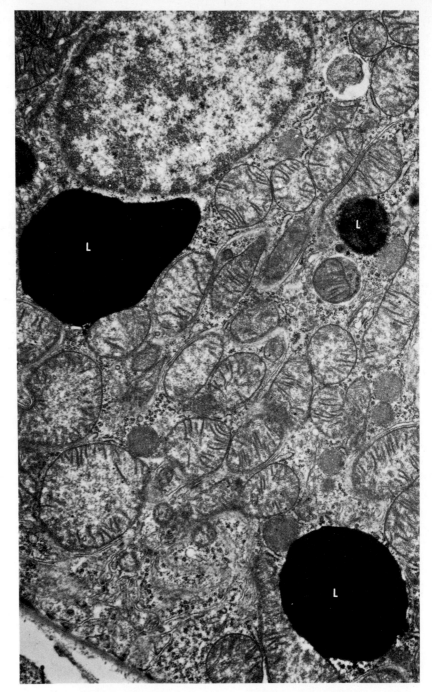

FIGURE VI–5. Electron micrograph showing a later stage after protein uptake by the proximal tubular cells. The horseradish peroxidase is now localized within lysosomes (L) deeper in the cells. × 11,700.

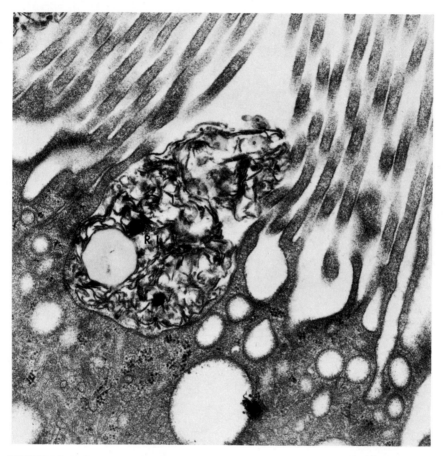

FIGURE VI–6. Electron micrograph showing the release of material from a residual lysosome (RL). The membrane surrounding the lysosome fuses with the cell membrane and the material from the residual lysosome (RL) moves into the tubular lumen. × 23,300.

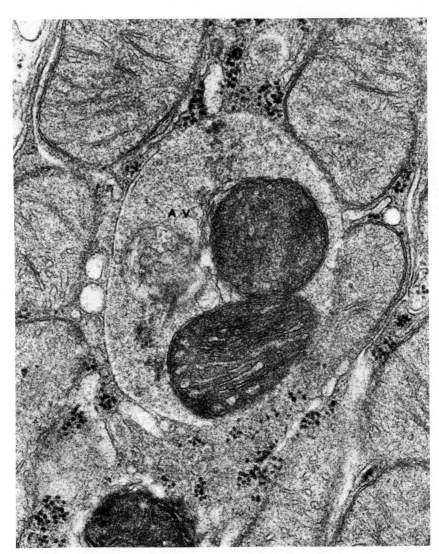

FIGURE VI–7. Electron micrograph showing an autophagic vacuole (AV) surrounded by a single membrane. The autophagic vacuole contains the remnants of two mitochondria in the process of being digested. × 49,800.

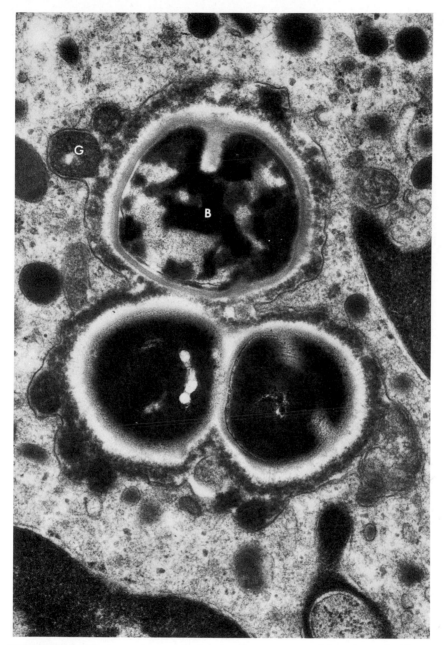

FIGURE VI–8. Electron micrograph showing the remnants of three bacteria (B) being digested within an autophagic vacuole of a polymorphonuclear leukocyte. The granules (G) normally seen within the cytoplasm of the leukocytes are releasing their contents into the autophagic vacuole. × 34,300.

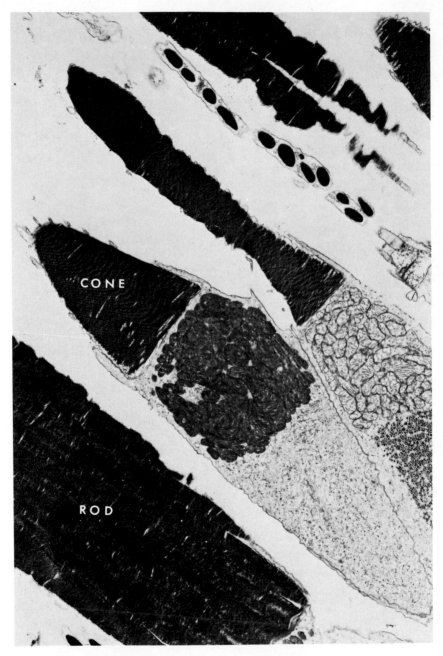

FIGURE VII–2. Electron micrograph showing part of a retina with an outer rod segment and an outer cone segment. × 6,300. Micrograph courtesy of Dr. Anita Hendrickson.

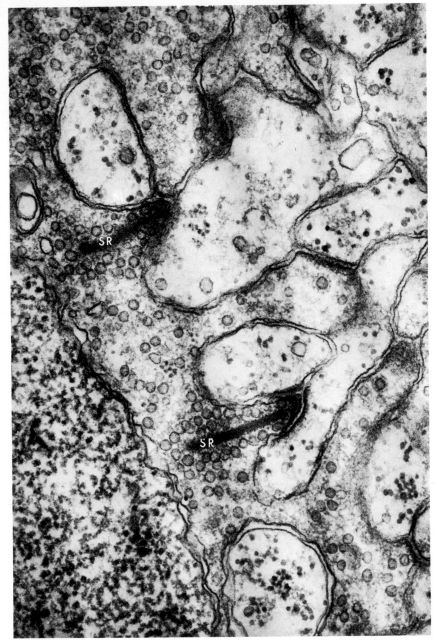

FIGURE VII–3. Electron micrograph showing a synapse between a photoreceptor and a bipolar cell. The photoreceptor contains two synaptic ribbons (SR). These are associated with vesicular structures. × 52,400. Micrograph courtesy of Dr. Anita Hendrickson.

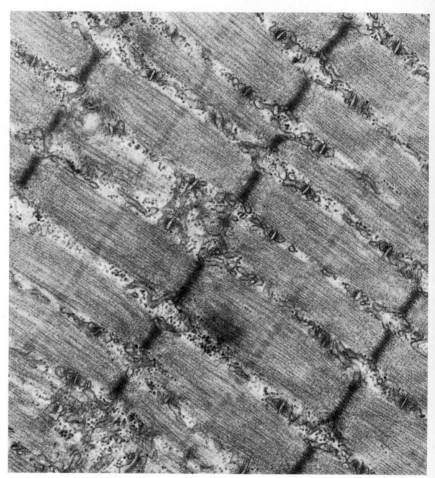

FIGURE VII–5. Electron micrograph showing part of the cytoplasm of a striated muscle cell. Parallel-oriented myofilaments comprise the longitudinal bundles called myofibrils. × 25,300.

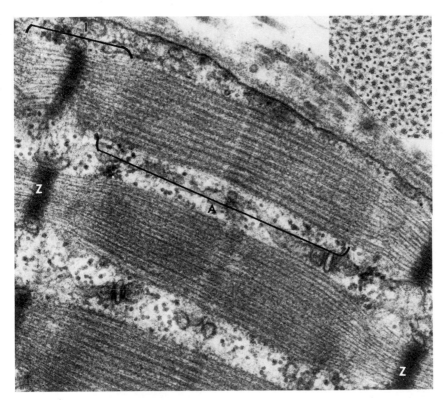

FIGURE VII–6. Electron micrograph showing the banding pattern of a striated muscle cell. The thick filaments comprise the *A* band, whereas thinner filaments comprise the *I* band and continue into the *A* zone. The *I* band is bisected by the *Z* line. The distance from one *Z* to the next *Z* is called a sarcomere. × 45,500. Inset: cross section of an *A* band showing the thick *A* filaments and surrounded by six thin *I* filaments. × 57,000.

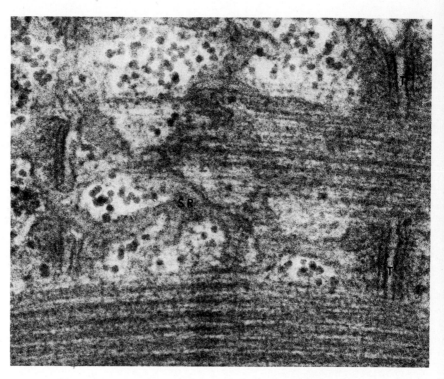

FIGURE VII–7. Electron micrograph showing a small section of the cytoplasm of striated muscle cell in which the sarcoplasmic reticulum (SR) can be seen. The sarcoplasmic reticulum comes into close associaton with the *T*-tubule. × 85,500.

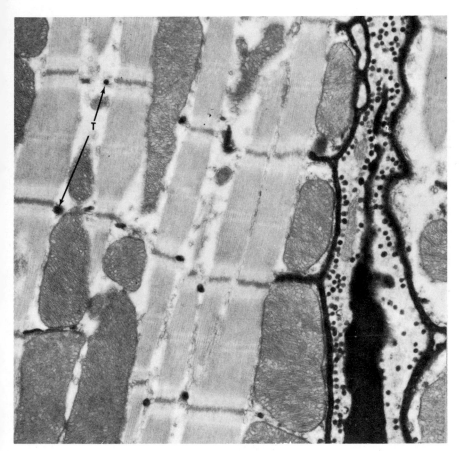

FIGURE VII–8. Electron micrograph showing the tracer horseradish peroxidase which appears dense in this picture. The tracer is seen deep in the *T*-tubule invaginations, indicating that they communicate with the extracellular space. The tracer is also seen within the lumen of the adjacent capillary as well as in vesicles and caveolae within the adjacent endothelial cell. Micrograph courtesy of Dr. M. J. Karnovsky. Reprinted by permission from *J. Gen. Physiol.*, 52 (1968), 64s–95s.

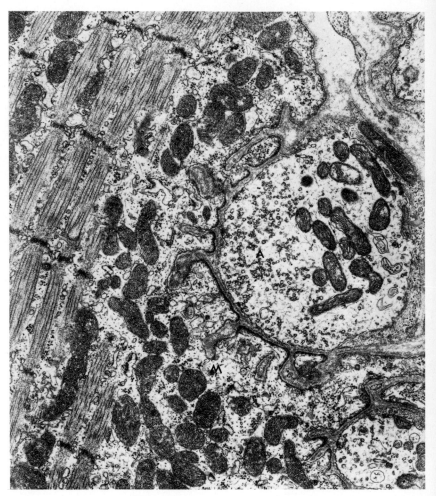

FIGURE VII–9. Electron micrograph showing a neuromuscular junction from a muscle located in the eye of a primate. The axon terminal (A) can be seen in a depression along the surface of the striated muscle cell (M). Micrograph courtesy of Miss Mary Cahill and Dr. Douglas Kelly. × 18,600.

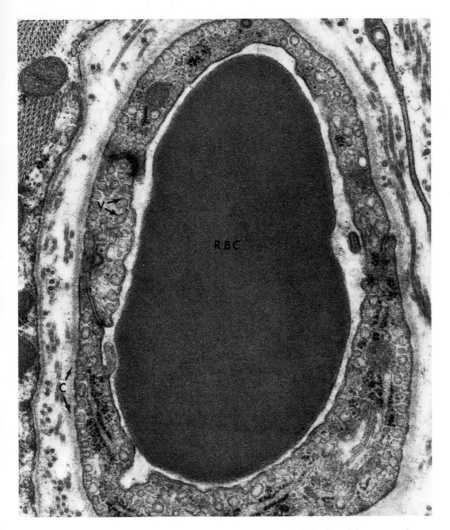

FIGURE VIII–1. Electron micrograph of a capillary which is lined by a continuous type of endothelium lacking fenestrae. This endothelium, however, contains caveolae (C) and vesicles (V). The lumen of this capillary contains a single red blood cell. × 27,400.

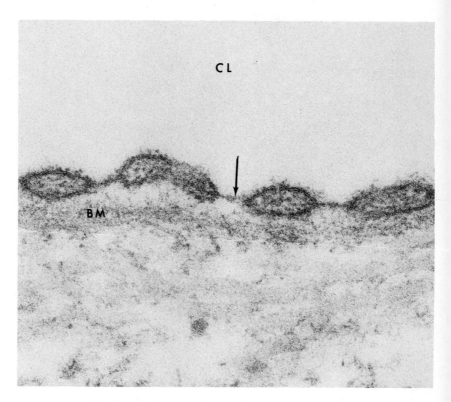

FIGURE VIII–2. Electron micrograph showing a small portion of the capillary endothelium from a fenestrated type of capillary. A capillary lumen (CL) is seen at the top of the picture. The small pores are each bridged by a narrow diaphragm (arrow). A thin basement membrane (BM) can be seen underlying the capillary. × 104,400.

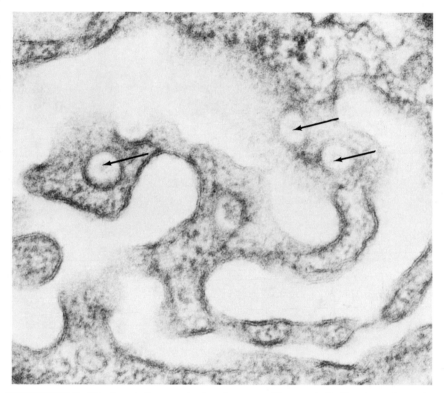

FIGURE VIII–3. Electron micrograph showing a capillary endothelium in surface view. From this angle, the central pore region shows increased density (arrows). × 104,400.

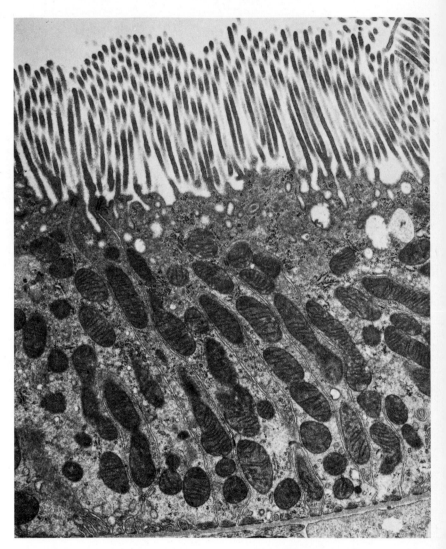

FIGURE VIII–4. Electron micrograph of a proximal convoluted tubular cell from a nephron. The cell is active in pumping ions and therefore contains many mitochondria. The mitochondria are aligned in such a manner that they lie adjacent to numerous lateral cell membranes formed from interdigitating processes of adjacent cells. × 10,400.

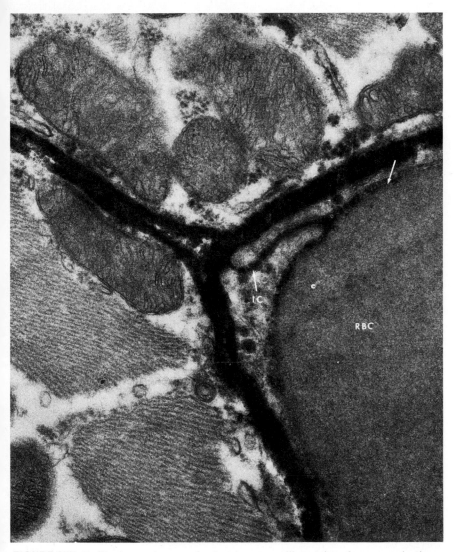

FIGURE VIII–5. Electron micrograph showing a capillary taken from muscle tissue. The capillary lumen contains a red blood cell (RBC). The tracer horseradish peoxidase can be seen in the layer between the red blood cell membrane and the lining endothelium (arrow). It can also be seen in the intercellular cleft (IC) between endothelial cells. × 113,600. Micrograph courtesy of Dr. M. J. Karnovsky. Reprinted by permission from *J. Cell Biol.* 35 (1967), 213.

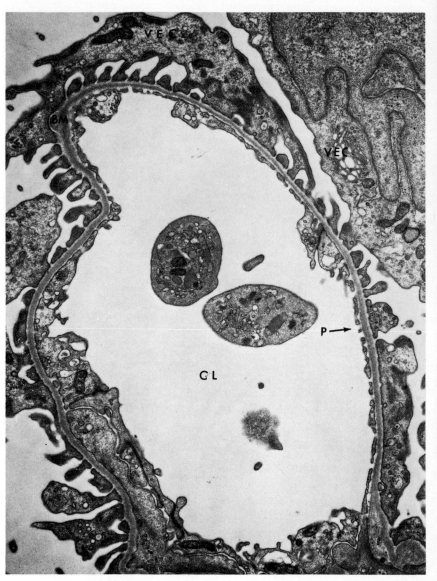

FIGURE VIII–6. Electron micrograph showing a capillary loop from a renal corpuscle of a rat kidney. Platelets lie within the capillary lumen (CL) surrounded by a thin layer of endothelium which is perforated by pores (P). A basement membrane (BM) lies between the endothelium and the processes of the visceral epithelial cells (VEC). The processes of the epithelial cells interdigitate along the basement membrane. × 6,200.

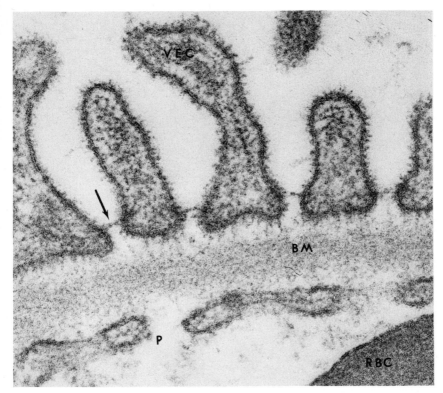

FIGURE VIII–7. Electron micrograph showing the filtration barrier of the renal corpuscle. A red blood cell (RBC) lies in the lumen of the capillary. The endothelial
cell is perforated by pores (P). A basement membrane (BM) lies between the capillary
endothelium and the processes of the visceral epithelial cell (VEC). A small filtration-slit
membrane (arrow) bridges the gap between adjacent processes. × 95,200.

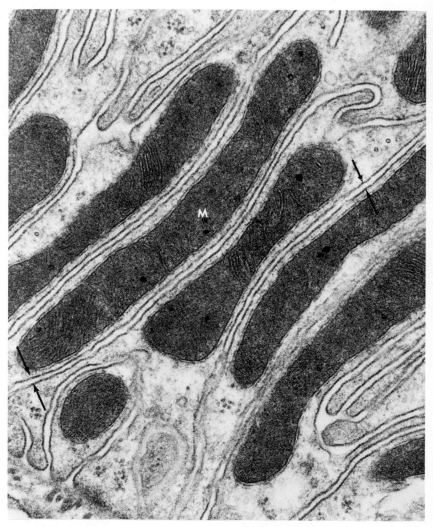

FIGURE VIII–8. Electron micrograph showing the basal region of a cell involved in the active transport of ions. The numerous mitochondria (M) are seen in close apposition to the lateral cell membranes (arrows) of adjacent interdigitating cells. × 39,200.

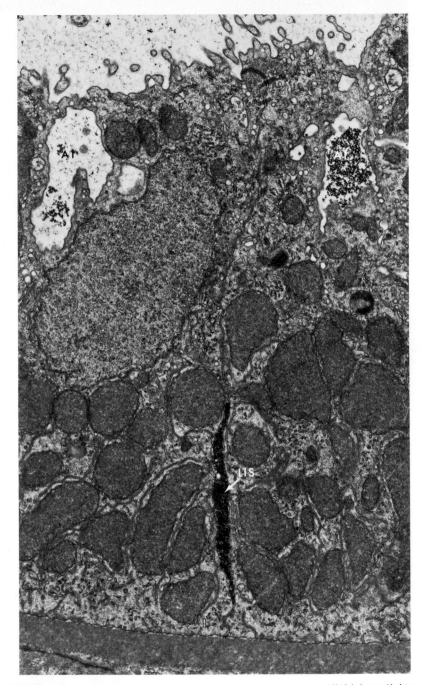

FIGURE VIII–11. Electron micrograph showing that when colloidal particles are injected retrograde up the ureter into the nephrons of intact flounder kidneys, these particles are taken up in apical invaginations (AI) and transported across the apical cell cytoplasm into the lateral intercellular spaces (LIS). × 13,200.

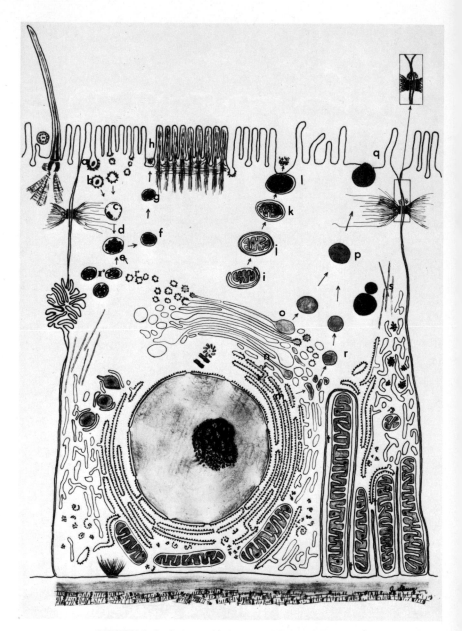

FIGURE S–1. Schematic drawing of a composite cell.

body portion of the amoeba flows into them, the organism moves forward by amoeboid movement. Some amoebae emit only a single, broad, blunt pseudopod, but others project many narrow branching ones. In order for an amoeba to manifest this kind of locomotion, it must have a solid surface to which it may adhere.

Amoeboid movement is related to changes in the amount of gelation within the ground substance (protoplasm) of the cell. These reversible changes from a liquid (sol) state to a semisolid (gel) state are known as sol–gel transformations. They probably represent the assembly of a temporary filamentous network within the cytoplasm that is capable of contraction. The detailed description of the advance of a single typical pseudopod is thought to be related to sol–gel reversibility. First, a clear outer ectoplasm expands near the tip of the advancing pseudopod. The ectoplasm appears to be stiff (plasma gel). The larger mass of the amoeba consists of a granular endoplasm. This endoplasm (plasma sol) breaks through the clear ectoplasmic cap and flows into it. The change from a gel to a sol state is explained according to the following theory: within the gel, chains of protein molecules are held together by cross-links.[16] Pressure, temperature, and ionic changes are thought to alter the degree of protein folding, thus changing the length of the protein chains. In gelled regions of the amoeba, long chains of protein molecules are believed to be unfolded and interrelated in such a way as to form a network. In sol areas of the protoplasm, globular protein molecules exist. A motive force within the amoeba causes the gel to "contract," and as it does so the protein chains fold to form globular protein molecules, resulting in a sol.

This explanation for the sol–gel changes that occur in amoeboid movement does not describe the source of the motive force that performs the work nor whether the mechanism is a "push" from the rear of the amoeba or a "pull" from the front. However, it appears that ATP plays a role in the process. It has been shown experimentally that the injection of ATP into amoebae causes their ectoplasmic gel to "contract" and liquify.[15] Many theories have been advanced to explain the mechanism of amoeboid movement,[1,15,16] but the process is still not well understood.*

CILIARY MOVEMENT

Cilia and flagella are motile eucaryotic cell processes. (Procaryotic or bacterial flagella are an entirely different organelle.) When a free cell

---

*A recent paper by T. D. Pollard and S. Ito [*J. Cell. Biol.*, 46 (1970), 267] utilizing extracts of *Amoeba proteus* cytoplasm suggest that the presence of 70-Å-unit and 160-Å-unit filaments may be necessary for movement. When ATP is added to the warmed extract, actin-like filaments 50 to 70 Å in diameter appear in conjunction with the increase in viscosity. Pollard and Ito propose that these filaments interact with the 160-Å-unit filaments constantly present to cause the contraction responsible for amoeboid movement.

bears one or a few of these long processes, they are frequently referred to as *flagella*.[11] Most sperm cells bear flagella. On the other hand, somewhat shorter, more numerous motile cell processes, having the same basic internal structure, are known as *cilia*. *Paramecium* is a protozoan whose surface bears hundreds of cilia. These cilia are used to propel the animal about in the water. Certain cells of higher animals also possess cilia. For example, epithelial cells lining the tracheal portion of the respiratory tract have parallel rows of cilia projecting from their luminal surfaces. The remarkable ability of cilia to beat rhythmically is well documented. All the cilia of a single cell can beat together, but more commonly, ciliary rows are activated in sequence giving the appearance of waves sweeping over the cell. The metachronal waves are rhythmic in occurrence and they are propagated in a given direction. Through this coordinated activity, ciliated cells lining the respiratory tract are able to move mucus and/or particulate matter away from the delicate tissues of the lung.

The movement of a cilium is related to its internal structure. When cut in cross section, most cilia display eleven internal fibrils (Fig. IV–10a). These are arranged in a 9 + 2 configuration: two fibrils—or more properly, microtubules—in the center and nine double fibrils evenly spaced in a circle around them. The ciliary microtubules are, like cytoplasmic microtubules, composed of subfilaments made up of a globular protein *tubulin*. Each of the outer nine doublets looks like a figure 8 with c-shaped arms projecting from the end of the doublet. An observer looking along a cilium from a base to the tip would see the arms projected clockwise.[5] Throughout the plant and animal kingdoms, cilia tend to possess this same basic internal structure. The basal bodies of cilia display specializations known as *striated rootlets*, which serve to anchor these motile processes to the cell cortex (Fig. IV–10b).

Recently a protein called *dynein* has been isolated from cilia;[14] it has ATPase activity. When dynein is experimentally removed from isolated preparations of cilia, the arms disappear from the outer doublets. Adding dynein again restores the arms to the doublet structures. Because of their enzymatic activity, the arms are thought to play a role in ciliary motility. Cilia whose membranes have been removed by certain chemical treatments will beat following the addition of ATP to a proper ionic environment. The cilium hydrolyzes the ATP in the beating process. Moreover, sperm tails, severed from their heads, will swim forward with their usual motion after such treatment.

Each cilium beats in a specific plane always oriented in the same direction. During the more rapid forward stroke, the cilium becomes stiff; during the slower recovery stroke, it becomes flexible somewhat like the arm stroke used in swimming the crawl. Several theories have been advanced to explain how the cilium accomplishes its whip-like movement. One theory proposes that the ciliary microtubules slide with respect to each other to produce bending. It does not solve the problem of how the dynein ATPase is involved in the production of this sliding, but at least it does appear to fit in with other evidence concerning cytoplasmic microtubules that suggests that they can move substances relative to themselves without substantially shortening by contraction. This theory is also attractive because it appears analogous in some ways to the well-established sliding filament theory of striated muscle contraction (see Chapter VII).[34]

MUSCULAR MOVEMENT

Muscle cells are highly specialized for movement. They have the ability to shorten in length when they contract. Because of their attachments to various tissues of the body, when these cells shorten in length they produce a variety of movements.

The shape and organization of skeletal muscle cells correlate well with their function. These long tube-like cells are filled with filaments aligned in a parallel array. The movement of these cytoplasmic filaments, with respect to one another, cause skeletal muscle cells to shorten in length. A single skeletal muscle cell, within the bundle of cells comprising a muscle, may be many centimeters long and extend the entire length of a muscle. Because skeletal muscle cells connect certain bones, these cells, by shortening in length, are able to cause movement at joints.

Smooth muscle cells often are arranged helically in sheets or layers within the walls of hollow structures such as arteries. In the gut, smooth muscle encircles the organ being arranged in an inner circular layer and outer longitudinal layer. The contraction of these cells ensheathing the gut allows mixing of the luminal contents with digestive enzymes and promotes movement of the contents along the digestive tract. Tiny smooth muscle cells are also attached to hair follicles in the skin. As these muscle cells contract, they pull at an angle upon the follicles and the hairs are made to stand erect, causing the appearance of "goose flesh." In animals with heavy coats of hair, this phenomenon provides a thicker layer of insulation against the cold. In most humans, however, it is of little use.

THE REGULATION OF CELL SIZE AND SHAPE

The complex factors which regulate cell size and shape are not well understood. It is clear, however, that both the nucleus and the cytoplasm are important in this respect.[38] Experiments with amoebae clearly indicate the interdependence of the nucleus and the cytoplasm.[7] Nuclei from one species of amoebae have been transferred into the cytoplasm of enucleated amoebae of other species. The cytoplasm caused an alteration in the size of the transplanted nuclei making them either larger or smaller than normal. Another interesting result was that the cytoplasm of the created hybrid amoebae dictated the shape of the pseudopods that were emitted. Nuclear size and the cell shape of these amoebae were therefore influenced by the cytoplasm.

The cytoplasm is also important in the inheritance of various characteristics related to cell shape in ciliate protozoa. Regeneration experiments with these organisms show that the cytoplasm signals the nucleus to begin synthesizing whatever is necessary in order to form a particular structure.[36]

The role of the nucleus in determining cell shape has been shown by hybrid grafts of the single-celled algae *Acetabularia*.[18] This large cell (3 to 4 centimeters long) looks like a mushroom with its cap, stalk, and rhizoid (root), which contains the nucleus. Cutting off the rhizoid with its nucleus leaves an enucleate *Acetabularia*. Grafting the rhizoid to another species of enucleate *Acetabularia* makes it possible to follow the effect of the nucleus on the hybrid. Such experiments demonstrate that the shape of the cap in these algae is under nuclear control. It is believed that the nucleus synthesizes chemical substances which direct the metabolic machinery within *Acetabularia* cytoplasm. As a result, when the original cap of the hybrid is cut off, a new cap shaped like that of the nuclear species is formed.

REFERENCES

[1] R. D. Allen, "A New Theory of Amoeboid Movement and Protoplasmic Streaming," *Exp. Cell Res. Suppl.*, 8 (1961), 17–31.

[2] O. Behnke, "Dynamics of Blood Platelet Microtubules," *J. Ultrastruct. Res.*, 20 (1967), 299–300.

[3] E. L. Benedetti and P. Emmelot, "Electron Microscopic Observations on Negatively Stained Plasma Membranes Isolated from Rat Liver," *J. Cell Biol.*, 26 (1965), 299–305.

[4] D. Bikle, L. G. Tielny, and K. R. Porter, "Microtubules and Pigment Migration in the Melanophores of *Fundulus heteroclitus* L.," *Protoplasma*, 61 (1966), 322–345.

[5] William Bloom and D. W. Fawcett, *A Textbook of Histology*, 9th ed. (Philadelphia: W. B. Saunders Co., 1968).

[6] R. E. Bulger and B. F. Trump, "Ca²⁺ and K⁺ Ion Effects on Ultrastructure of Isolated Flounder Kidney Tubules," *J. Ultrastruct. Res.*, 28 (1969), 301–319.

[7] J. F. Danielli, "The Cell-to-Cell Transfer of Nuclei in Amoebae and a Comprehensive Cell Theory," *Ann. N. Y. Acad. Sci.*, 78 (1959), 675–687.

[8] M. M. Dewey and Lloyd Barr, "Intercellular Connection Between Smooth Muscle Cells: The Nexus," *Science*, 137 (1962), 670–672.

[9] M. M. Dewey and Lloyd Barr, "Structure of Vertebrate Intestinal Smooth Muscle," in *Handbook of Physiology*, C. F. Code, ed., Vol. IV: Motility, Section 6: Alimentary Canal (Washington, D.C.: American Physiological Society, 1968), 1629–1654.

[10] M. G. Farquhar and G. E. Palade, "Junctional Complexes in Various Epithelia," *J. Cell Biol.*, 17 (1963), 375–412.

[11] D. W. Fawcett, *The Cell: Its Organelles and Inclusions* (Philadelphia: W. B. Saunders Co., 1966), 423.

[12]D. W. Fawcett and Frank Witebsky, "Observations on the Ultrastructure of Nucleated Erythrocytes and Thrombocytes, with Particular Reference to the Structural Basis of their Discoidal Shape," *Z. Zellforsch. Mikr. Anat.,* 62 (1964), 785–806.

[13]Y. C. B. Fung and P. Tong, "Theory of the Sphering of Red Blood Cells," *Biophys. J.,* 8 (1968), 175–198.

[14]I. R. Gibbons and A. J. Rowe, "Dynein: A Protein with Adenosine Triphosphatase Activity from Cilia," *Science,* 149 (1965), 424–426.

[15]R. J. Goldacre, "The Role of the Cell Membrane in the Locomotion of Amoebae, and the Source of the Motive Force and its Control by Feedback," *Exp. Cell Res. Suppl.,* 8 (1961), 1–16.

[16]R. J. Goldacre and I. J. Lorch, "Folding and Unfolding of Protein Molecules in Relation to Cytoplasmic Streaming, Amoeboid Movement and Osmotic Work," *Nature,* 166 (1950), 497–500.

[17]Lorna Green, "Mechanism of Movements of Granules in Melanocytes of *Fundulus heteroclitus,*" *Proc. Nat. Acad. Sci.,* 59 (1968), 1179–1186.

[18]J. Hämmerling, "Nucleo-Cytoplasmic Relationships in the Development of *Acetabularia,*" *Int. Rev. Cytol.,* 2 (1953), 475–498.

[19]H. Hartridge, "Shape of Red Blood Corpuscles," *J. Physiol.,* 53 (1919–1920), lxxxi.

[20]R. M. Hays, Bayla Singer, and Sasha Malamed, "The Effect of Calcium Withdrawal on the Structure and Function of the Toad Bladder," *J. Cell Biol.,* 25 (1965), 195–208.

[21]Tom Humphreys, "Chemical Dissolution and *in Vitro* Reconstruction of Sponge Cell Adhesions. I. Isolation and Functional Demonstration of the Components Involved," *Dev. Biol.,* 8 (1963), 27–47.

[22]H. S. Jacob, "Annotation: Dysfunction of the Red Blood Cell Membrane in Hereditary Spherocytosis," *Brit. J. Haemat.,* 14 (1968), 99–104.

[23]M. J. Karnovsky, "The Ultrastructural Basis of Capillary Permeability Studied with Peroxidase as a Tracer," *J. Cell Biol.,* 35 (1967), 213–236.

[24]D. E. Kelly, "Fine Structure of Desmosomes, Hemidesmosomes, and an Adepidermal Globular Layer in Developing Newt Epidermis," *J. Cell Biol.,* 28 (1966), 51–72.

[25]H. Lehmann and R. G. Huntsman, "Why Are Red Cells the Shape They Are? The Evolution of the Human Red Cell," in *Functions of the Blood,* R. G. MacFarlane and A. H. T. Robb-Smith, eds. (New York: Academic Press Inc., 1961), 73–148.

[26]W. R. Loewenstein and Yoshinobo Kanno, "Studies on an Epithelial (Gland) Cell Junction. I. Modifications of Surface Membrane Permeability," *J. Cell Biol.,* 22 (1964), 565–586.

[27]B. W. Payton, M. V. L. Bennett, and G. D. Pappas, "Permeability and Structure of Junctional Membranes at an Electronic Synapse," *Science,* 166 (1969), 1641–1643.

[28]L. D. Peachey, "Electron Microscopic Observatrions on the Accumulation of Divalent Cations in Intramitochondrial Granules," *J. Cell Biol.,* 20 (1964), 95–111.

[29]K. R. Porter, "Cytoplasmic Microtubules and Their Functions," in *Principles of Biomolecular Organization,* G. E. W. Wolstenholme and Maeve O'Connor, eds., Ciba Found., Gen. Symp. (Boston: Little, Brown and Co., 1966), 308–356.

[30]T. S. Reese and M. J. Karnovsky, "Fine Structural Localization of a Blood-Brain Barrier to Exogenous Peroxidase," *J. Cell Biol.,* 34 (1967), 207–217.

[31]J. P. Revel and M. J. Karnovsky, "Hexagonal Array of Subunits in Intercellular Junctions of the Mouse Heart and Liver," *J. Cell Biol.,* 33 (1967), C7–C12.

[32]J. D. Robertson "The Occurrence of a Subunit Pattern in the Unit Membranes of Club Endings in Mauthner Cell Synapses in Goldfish Brains," *J. Cell Biol.,* 19 (1963), 201–221.

[33]M. A. Rudzinska, "The Fine Structure and Function of the Tentacle in *Tokophrya infusionum,*" *J. Cell Biol.,* 25 (1965), 459–477.

[34]Peter Satir, "Studies on Cilia. III. Further Studies on the Cilium Tip and a 'Sliding Filament' Model of Ciliary Motility," *J. Cell Biol.,* 39 (1968), 77–94.

[35] A. W. Sedar and J. G. Forte, "Effects of Calcium Depletion on the Junctional Complex Between Oxyntic Cells of Gastric Glands," *J. Cell Biol.*, 22 (1964), 173–188.

[36] Vance Tartar, *Biology of Stentor* (New York: Pergamon Press, Inc., 1961).

[37] L. G. Tilney, Yukio Hiramoto, and Douglas Marsland, "Studies on the Microtubules in Heliozoa. III. A Pressure Analysis of the Role of These Structures in the Formation and Maintenance of the Axopodia of *Actinosphaerium nucleofilum* (Barrett)," *J. Cell Biol.*, 29 (1966), 77–95.

[38] R. J. C. Harris, ed., "The Relationship between Nucleus and Cytoplasm," *Exp. Cell Res. Suppl.*, 6 (Proc. Symp. Belgium, June 1958) (New York: Academic Press Inc., 1959).

[39] R. I. Weed and C. F. Reed, "Membrane Alterations Leading to Red Cell Destruction," *Amer. J. Med.*, 41 (1966), 681–698.

[40] Joseph Wiener, David Spiro, and W. R. Loewenstein, "Studies on an Epithelial (Gland) Cell Junction. II. Surface Structure," *J. Cell Biol.*, 22 (1964), 587–598.

V

CELLULAR
MACHINERY
IN ACTION:
How Cells
Manufacture Products

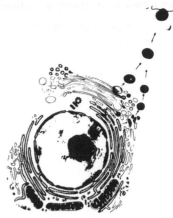

Cells manufacture a variety of different substances. Although most cells contain the same organelles (i.e., endoplasmic reticulum, Golgi apparatus, and so forth), their products reflect particular lines of specialization. For example, some cells of the intestinal epithelium synthesize mucus, endocrine gland cells manufacture hormones, while those comprising the salivary glands and pancreas produce digestive enzymes. These different secretory products are synthesized in various ways by these cell types. This chapter follows the manufacture of a few secretory products, tracing their synthesis in relation to various parts of the cytoplasmic machinery.

Although the specific chemical compounds secreted by cells differ, each falls into one or more of the major classes of compounds synthesized by cells: proteins, lipids, or carbohydrates. These macromolecular substances play many important roles in a variety of biological functions.

Proteins are perhaps the most important single group of macromolecules produced by cells. Not only do they provide the cell and its organelles with structural components, but as enzymes, they are essential in metabolism and transport processes. In addition, as antibodies, proteins are important in providing an immune defense mechanism, protecting the body against the invasion of harmful bacteria and other organisms (and substances) which are antigenic.

Lipids comprise a portion of cell membranes and provide an important source of metabolic energy. When stored as fat deposits, lipids also insulate the body against cold.

Carbohydrates are a major source of cellular energy. They combine with other chemical compounds such as proteins to form mucopoly-saccharides which comprise a large portion of the connective tissue matrix. The external surface of most cell membranes is coated by muco-polysaccharides, and these macromolecules have been credited with providing cells such as red blood cells with their antigenicity.

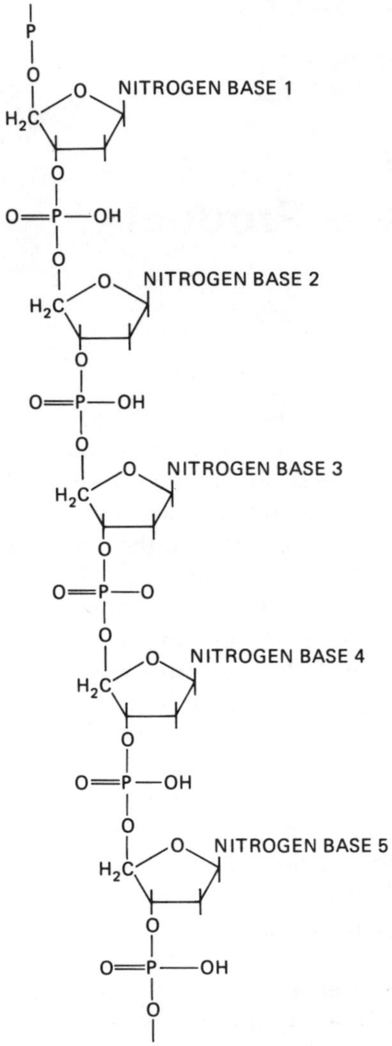

FIGURE V–1. The molecular "backbone" of the DNA molecule is composed of alternating phosphate and sugar residues. Nitrogen-containing bases are substituted on the sugar moieties.

PROTEIN SYNTHESIS

How do cells synthesize and release their many different chemical substances? Proteins manufactured by cells provide us with a well-studied example. The steps involved in protein synthesis have been elucidated only in the last 10 to 15 years. [1,27,29] They include the following: information coded in deoxyribonucleic acid (DNA) is first *transcribed* into the "language" of ribonucleic acid (RNA). The RNA then serves to *translate* this message by synthesizing protein molecules which correspond to those originally specified by the DNA. In order to understand these major steps better, it is necessary to look more closely at each part of the process.

The genetic information of an organism is contained within DNA. The large DNA macromolecule consists of four nitrogen-containing bases (adenine, thymine, cytosine, and guanine). These bases project from a molecular "backbone" that is composed of alternating phosphate and sugar residues (Fig. V–1). The phosphate-sugar-base moiety is known as a nucleotide. The DNA in most cells exists as two long strands of nucleotides which are intertwined to form a double helix (Fig. V–2). [9] The two strands of DNA are held together in a very precise manner, by hydrogen bonding between their complementary base pairs. For each adenine in one chain of the DNA double helix, a thymine exists opposite it in the corresponding chain; and for each cytosine, a guanine is present in the opposite strand (i.e., the bases are complementary). The genetic

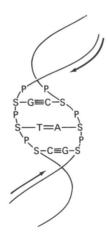

FIGURE V–2. Diagram showing the double helical structure of DNA with hydrogen bonds existing between complementary base pairs. Each adenine in one chain of the DNA double helix is bonded to a thymine in the corresponding chain, and each cytosine to a guanine.

code resides in the sequence of these four bases. During transcription of one DNA strand into the language of a messenger RNA (mRNA), complementary base pairing occurs. For every cytosine in DNA a guanine is placed into the mRNA; and for each guanine, a cytosine appears in the mRNA strand. However, for adenine, a uracil base is substituted in the mRNA, since RNA molecules do not contain thymine. The mRNA strand thus reflects the specific DNA that produced it, and as "messenger" it moves into the cytoplasm with the necessary information for protein synthesis. (Most of the work on RNA has been done utilizing bacterial systems and it is as yet unclear just how much of what has been learned there applies to mammalian cells.)

The four bases, adenine, uracil, cytosine, and guanine (A, U, C, and G, respectively), are thereby arranged in specific sequences along the strand of mRNA. Their particular arrangement along mRNA makes up the code for the twenty amino acids that constitute protein molecules. Three of these bases in sequence (a triplet) are required in order to specify one amino acid in the process of protein synthesis. For example, the mRNA "word" UUU (from the bases AAA in DNA) is translated as the amino acid "phenylalanine" during synthesis. However, the strand of mRNA alone cannot recognize amino acids and order them into polypeptides. Its role is to act as a template, or instruction tape, spelling out the particular amino acids which are to be placed into the growing polypeptide.

In addition to the instructions provided by mRNA, a smaller kind of RNA called transfer RNA (tRNA) is essential in the process of polypeptide synthesis. This type of RNA is also referred to as soluble RNA (sRNA), because after cells have been subjected to intense ultracentrifugation for many hours, sRNA remains in the supernatant fraction. Each tRNA binds specifically to a particular amino acid. An enzyme enables tRNA to attach itself to that amino acid (AA), thus forming an "activated" tRNA–AA complex. The portion (or end) of the tRNA that is not attached to the amino acid has a special sequence of three unpaired bases (cytosine, guanine, uracil, or adenine in any order). These three unpaired tRNA bases (which constitute an *anticodon*) recognize an appropriate triplet of bases along the mRNA strand (a *codon*). Complementary base pairing, via the formation of hydrogen bonds, takes place between the anticodon of the tRNA bearing its amino acid, and the codon of the mRNA (Fig. V–3).[29] As a result of this process a particular amino acid is put into its place in the polypeptide. Additional amino acids are sequentially placed into position and a special enzyme links them into the growing polypeptide chain by forming peptide bonds.

This ordering of amino acids into polypeptides (protein synthesis) occurs in relation to ribosomal particles within the cell. The ribosomes comprise yet another fraction of cellular RNA. Usually five or more ribosomes

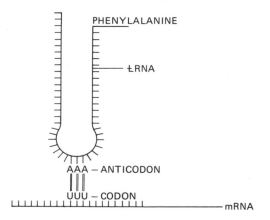

PHENYLALANINE

tRNA

AAA – ANTICODON

UUU – CODON

mRNA

FIGURE V–3. Complementary base pairing also occurs between mRNA and "activated" tRNA–AA complex.

are found aggregated, presumably along a strand of mRNA, forming a polysome.[29] These ribosome complexes are the sites where amino acids are assembled into polypeptide chains. Each ribosome is a particle composed of RNA and protein. It measures approximately 150 to 250 Ångströms in diameter and consists of two subunits. When subjected to ultracentrifugation, in media of low magnesium ion concentration, the ribosome can be dissociated into its two parts. An intact ribosome has a sedimentation constant (S) of 80 S and when dissociated, two subunits (one 40 S and one 60 S) are obtained (Fig. V–4). The smaller subunit of the ribosome appears to bind the mRNA[33] and the "activated" tRNA–AA complexes.[20] In animal cells which contain rough-surfaced endoplasmic reticulum, it is the larger subunit that sits on the membrane.[31] Protein synthesized by these ribosomes for export appears to be released through the membranes into the cisternae of the endoplasmic reticulum. Although the molecular structure of the ribosome is not understood, recent experimental evidence indicates that it possesses two different sites for the attachment of tRNAs.[8] The first site, known as the amino acid site, is thought to receive and position the "activated" tRNA–AA complex. The second site, known as the peptide site, holds the tRNA while a

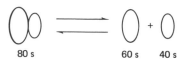

80 s   60 s   40 s

FIGURE V–4. The intact ribosome has a sedimentation constant of 80 S units which, when dissociated, forms two subunits (one 40 S and one 60 S).

peptide bond is formed between its attached amino acid and that of the last amino acid on the growing polypeptide chain (Fig. V–5).

In summary, information is stored in the DNA molecule, being coded in the arrangement of the purine and pyrimidine bases which exist in the long macromolecular strand. During cell division each strand of the DNA double helix can serve as a template for the formation of a new DNA molecule. Because complementary base pairing occurs, each newly formed DNA double helix will have the same coded information as that in the original DNA. Under the proper conditions, a portion of the DNA strand can also serve as a template for the formation of mRNA molecules. The mRNA may be thought of as an instruction tape. It moves into the cytoplasm of the cell and there it functions as a template for aligning amino acids. The ribosomes (polysomes) read its contained code and synthesize the protein that has been dictated by DNA. Ribosomes apparently have two sites (an amino acid site, and a peptide site) that accommodate tRNA molecules. An "activated" tRNA–AA complex arrives at the amino acid site and places its attached amino acid into position. As the ribosomes and the mRNA move with respect to one another, this amino acid is transferred to the peptide site. Here an enzyme forms a peptide bond and the amino acid becomes part of the growing polypeptide chain. Protein synthesis therefore requires three classes of RNA molecules—messenger RNA, transfer RNA, and ribosomal RNA—as well as amino acids and the necessary enzymes for each step. The molecular mechanisms involved in the steps from DNA to RNA (transcription) and from RNA into the finished polypeptide chain (translation) are beginning to be understood (Fig. V–6).

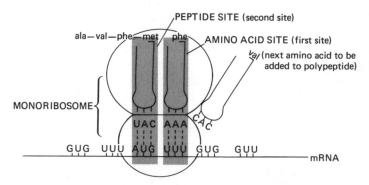

FIGURE V–5. The two subunits of the ribosome are thought to be related to a strand of mRNA. The ribosome has an amino acid site and a peptide site. The "activated" tRNA–AA complex, which is coded for in the mRNA, arrives at the amino acid site of the ribosome. This amino acid is then transferred to the peptide site where the peptide bond is formed and the newly arrived amino acid becomes part of the growing polypeptide chain.

DNA – – – – – –transcription– – – – – ⟶ RNA – – – – –translation– – – – ⟶Protein

messenger
transfer
ribosomal

FIGURE V–6. Diagram showing the overall process of protein synthesis from DNA to the protein.

However, knowledge about the underlying mechanisms whereby cells manufacture substances is far from complete and many questions of major significance remain to be answered.[10] For example, how is the transcription of DNA regulated? Is the amount of a particular protein synthesized by a cell related to the number of mRNA copies produced by its DNA? What determines the lifetime of a mRNA molecule, and in what form is mRNA transferred from the nucleus to the cytoplasm? Do mRNA templates differ in their rates of protein synthesis and if so, what determines this variation?

The mechanisms of initiation and termination of protein synthesis are presently being investigated. In the bacterium *Escherichia coli* it has been found that a variant of the amino acid methionine is responsible for beginning the synthesis of a protein.[8] This variant amino acid (formyl methionine) has a formyl group substituted for one of the hydrogen atoms usually present in the terminal amino group of methionine (Fig. V–7). It is thought that the formyl group changes the configuration of the amino acid and allows it to move directly to the peptide site of the ribosome. It is thus able to initiate the synthesis of a polypeptide chain. Although formyl methionine is able to begin the synthesis of a protein in microorganisms, nothing is known about the mechanisms responsible for initiating this process in higher animals. The termination of protein synthesis in certain bacteria is associated with particular codon triplets. Whenever three bases occur in the specific sequences UAA, UAG, or UGA, synthesis stops and the polypeptide is released from the ribosome.[11] Recent evidence indicates that a protein-releasing factor is also required for the release of a newly formed peptide.[5]

$$H—N—H$$
$$CH_3—S—CH_2—CH_2—\overset{|}{\underset{|}{C}}—COOH$$
$$H$$

METHIONINE

$$H—N—C\overset{O}{\underset{H}{\diagup}}$$
$$CH_3—S—CH_2—CH_2—\overset{|}{\underset{|}{C}}—COOH$$
$$H$$

FORMYL METHIONINE

FIGURE V–7. Diagram comparing methionine with formyl methionine.

Not only is the specific chemical nature of the cell product determined by the specialized cell in which it is manufactured, but the location and fate of the product are determined as well. This can clearly be shown for newly synthesized polypeptides (or proteins). In cells where the polysomes lie free in the cytoplasm (i.e., red blood cells) the synthesized protein is released into the cytoplasmic matrix where it becomes functional. A good example of this is the protein hemoglobin, which is contained in mammalian red blood cells, and which carries molecular oxygen to various cells of the body. In cells where polysomes are found attached to intracellular membranes, forming the rough-surfaced endoplasmic reticulum (for example, exocrine pancreas cells), the newly synthesized protein is usually exported from the cell. As it is released from the polysome, the protein is transferred into the cisternae of the endoplasmic reticulum. Following intracellular transport, it is ultimately discharged from the cell. In general, cells which synthesize protein for export have an abundance of rough-surfaced endoplasmic reticulum, while those engaged in the synthesis of protein for their own use contain many free polysomes in their cytoplasm.

One of the most elegant series of studies involving the synthesis, intracellular transport, and storage of proteins describes the production of digestive enzymes in the exocrine cells of the pancreas. The pancreas is a large gland having a duct which leads into the lumen of the digestive tract. This organ produces hydrolytic digestive enzymes which are released into the lumen of the intestine, where they function in the breakdown of food products. Dr. G. E. Palade and his collaborators have used the techniques of electron microscopy, biochemical fractionation, and radioautography to arrive at a detailed picture of protein synthesis and secretion.[7,14,15,16,17]

The first cellular machinery used by exocrine pancreas cells is the rough-surfaced endoplasmic reticulum (Fig. V–8). The ribosomes attached to the membranes of this organelle align and incorporate amino acids into protein. The newly synthesized protein is then transferred into the cisternae of the rough-surfaced endoplasmic reticulum. Movement within these cisternae brings the protein to the region of the cell where the Golgi apparatus (Fig. V–9) is located. The protein is then transported out of the cisternae of the endoplasmic reticulum in small vesicles formed by an evagination of the cisternal wall. These isolated protein-containing vesicles fuse with condensing vacuoles of the Golgi complex (Fig. V–10). Within these Golgi vacuoles the protein becomes concentrated and condensed (packaged) into zymogen granules. You will recall that the word zymogen designates an inactive form of the enzyme, indicating that it must be altered chemically or enzymatically in order to have enzymatic activity. The zymogen granules, containing their digestive enzymes, are stored in the exocrine cells of the pancreas (Fig. V–11). As more and more newly synthesized granules gradually move away from the Golgi region, they begin to accumulate in the apical region of the cells. The zymogen granules remain stored in the cells in this manner until hormones (associated with the digestion of particular foodstuffs) signal for their discharge. *Pancreozymin* is a hormone released from cells lining the duodenal portion of the intestine. It has been shown to trigger the release of zymogen granules in isolated preparations of pancreas.[12] The mechanism of granule release involves fusion of the membrane surrounding the zymogen granule with the cell membrane (Fig. V–12). Then, by a process of exocytosis, the digestive enzymes contained within the granule are released from the cell. Occasionally zymogen granules coalesce with other granules that have already fused with the cell membrane, perhaps permitting a more rapid release of their contents.

LIPID SYNTHESIS

Lipid metabolism has been studied quite extensively, but the role that cell organelles play in the synthesis of this group of substances still remains uncertain. Much of the lipid present in animal tissues comes from dietary intake. After leaving the stomach, lipids enter the lumen of the small intestine in the form of tiny droplets, which consist primarily of unhydrolyzed triglycerides. These fat droplets are emulsified by the action of bile salts. A lipase (an enzyme released from the pancreas in the manner just described) also acts upon this emulsified lipid, hydrolyzing its triglycerides to monoglycerides and free fatty acids. The monoglycerides and free fatty acids, in combination with bile salts, form negatively charged polymolecular aggregates, called micelles.[4] Micelles measure approximately 50 to 100 Ångström units in diameter and still contain small quantities of diglycerides and triglycerides. In the form of micelles, the monoglycerides and free fatty acids are transported along the intestine to the upper portion of the jejunum, where fat absorption occurs. Whether the intact micelles penetrate the intestinal cells, or whether their monoglycerides and free fatty acids are released at the cell membrane and absorbed by selective diffusion, is still uncertain. However, the uptake process itself has been shown experimentally to be independent of an energy-supplying system.[18]

The extent to which triglycerides are broken down, before being taken into absorptive cells, still remains a subject of controversy. Some investigators believe that intestinal cells take up at least some of the unhydrolyzed fat droplets by pinocytosis.[24] In experiments where animals fed fat, small membranous invaginations between the apical microvilli of the intestinal cells were observed to contain fat droplets. These were presented as evidence that lipid droplets were engulfed and transported into the cell. Later in time the endoplasmic reticulum displayed fat droplets and the theory was advanced that the pinocytotic vesicles fused with the membranes of the endoplasmic reticulum, thereby transferring the fat into the cisternae of this organelle. Although in some cases pinocytosis may play a role in fat uptake, more recent experimental evidence indicates that this process is not a major mechanism whereby fat is absorbed.[25] It has been shown that fat absorption continues under conditions that inhibit energy-requiring processes.[18] Since pinocytosis appears to depend upon energy, it cannot be responsible for this continued fat uptake. It seems most likely that the monoglycerides and free fatty acids, which result from hydrolysis in the gut lumen, diffuse through the microvillous membrane and into the cytoplasm of the intestinal absorptive cell.

Electron microscopical studies indicate that the endoplasmic reticulum undergoes a marked alteration during fat absorption.[6] The smooth-surfaced endoplasmic reticulum in the apical region of the absorptive cell accumulates lipid droplets at a rapid rate. It appears that its membranes pick up the monoglycerides and free fatty acids and resynthesize them into triglycerides, since biochemical studies show that the enzymes for triglyceride synthesis are localized in the microsome fraction of the cell. This fraction contains both rough- and smooth-surfaced endoplasmic reticulum as well as the Golgi apparatus. In electron micrographs, lipid is found much more frequently in the smooth-surfaced endoplasmic reticulum than it is in the rough-surfaced endoplasmic reticulum.[6] Moreover, the rough-surfaced endoplasmic reticulum appears to diminish and the smooth-surfaced endoplasmic reticulum appears to increase during the process of fat absorption. Additional evidence for the smooth-surfaced endoplasmic reticulum being the primary site for triglyceride resynthesis comes from experimental work with puromycin[19] and carbon tetrachloride.[32] When administered to an animal, these agents inhibit protein synthesis by disrupting the rough-surfaced endoplasmic reticulum, but they do not interfere with the synthesis of triglycerides.

As triglycerides are resynthesized within the cell, they become coated by protein and form insoluble droplets, called *chylomicrons*. Chylomicrons measure approximately 0.1 to 1.5 microns and are the final products of lipid absorption and resynthesis by cells. They are the form in which lipids are exported from intestinal cells. Their protein coating facilitates and makes possible the transport of large quantities of water-insoluble lipids in an aqueous extracellular environment. Although the mechanism of chylomicron release is unclear, it appears likely that by a reverse pinocytotic process (exocytosis) at the lateral cell surfaces, these particles are delivered into the intercellular spaces. From here the chylomicrons move into the extracellular space, then cross the basement membrane underlying the cells and into nearby *lacteals*. (Lacteals are blind lymph capillaries that are beginning channels leading into the larger ducts which comprise the lymphatic system.) From lymphatic channels the tiny fat-containing particles empty into the bloodstream to be carried via the circulation to cells, such as those of the liver and heart, throughout the body, where they become metabolized.

A lipid droplet may remain free in the cytoplasm of the cell as stored lipid, or in combination with protein it may be exported from the cell as lipoprotein. Lipoproteins are synthesized in the liver and released into the circulation where they comprise a good percentage of the plasma lipids. Within the liver cell, proteins synthesized by the ribosomes of the rough-surfaced endoplasmic reticulum are transferred from its cisternae into that of the smooth-surfaced endoplasmic reticulum, where they become linked to lipid.[19] Occasionally in liver cells, the Golgi complex also reveals fat particles. Since some lipoproteins contain carbohydrate groupings (for example, glycolipoproteins), it is believed that the Golgi complex participates in their formation by synthesizing carbohydrate moieties and attaching them to the lipoprotein.[19] In such cases the synthetic pathway would include movement of lipid from the smooth-surfaced endoplasmic reticulum into the Golgi region. From the endoplasmic reticulum (or the Golgi complex) membrane-bound structures containing lipid particles are budded off. These vesicles move to the surface of the cell, where, by a mechanism of exocytosis, they release their contained lipoproteins.

COMPLEX CARBOHYDRATE SYNTHESIS

In addition to proteins and lipids, polysaccharides constitute a third major category of substances synthesized by cells. Among these are the "complex carbohydrates," which include glycoproteins, mucopolysaccharides, glycolipids, and glycogen. The goblet cells of the colon, which produce a carbohydrate-rich mucus secretion, have been studied most extensively (Fig. V–13). These cells are goblet shaped, the bowl portion being filled with granules of mucous. Electron microscopical radioautography indicates that the mucous granules are synthesized in the following manner.[21] Amino acids in the capillaries of the intestine enter the goblet cells, where they are synthesized into proteins in the rough-surfaced endoplasmic reticulum in a manner analogous to that described for the pancreas. The newly synthesized proteins are then transported to the Golgi complex, which synthesizes carbohydrates from simple sugars and links them to the incoming proteins. Sulfate is added to the carbohydrate part of the new glycoprotein within the Golgi complex.[23] As the glycoprotein product accumulates, it distends the Golgi saccules, transforming them into completed mucous globules. The packaged mucous globules migrate to the apical region of the cell, where they can be released into the intestinal lumen.

The goblet cells are not the only cells which use the Golgi complex as a synthetic organelle for complex carbohydrates. Pancreas, epididymis, liver, and other intestinal cells also incorporate radioactive precursors of glycoproteins and mucopolysaccharides in their Golgi complexes.[22]

The outer surface of most, if not all, cell membranes have a carbohydrate-rich coating *(glycocalyx)*.[3] In absorptive cells this surface coating is clearly visible as a layer of fuzz, continuous with (or part of) the outer membrane (Fig. IV–7). It has been thought that this layer represents an accumulation of adsorbed mucus which has been elaborated by other cells. In order to determine the site where this carbohydrate-rich coat is synthesized, a series of autoradiographic studies was undertaken.[13] The incorporation of radioactive labeled precursors (such as mannose-^{3}H, sulfate-^{35}S and glucosamine-^{14}C) into mucopolysaccharides was followed in isolated intestinal absorptive cells.[13] By observation of electron micrographs the labeled substances were first localized in the Golgi region of the cells. With time, the label moved apically and became localized over the carbohydrate-rich coat (fuzz) of the microvillous border. Exactly how the surface coat material is transported from the Golgi complex to the cell surface is not yet clear, but it is evident that the cells themselves synthesize this layer.[13]

Cartilage is a type of connective tissue that helps to form and maintain the structure of the ear, nose, trachea, larynx, and other parts of the body. The resilience of cartilage is largely due to its matrix, which contains a significant amount of mucopolysaccharide material closely related to collagen fibrils. Cartilage cells synthesize these complex carbohydrates and experimental studies indicate that the Golgi apparatus plays a role in their manufacture.[23] Moreover, in differentiating cartilage, precursors of the extracellular collagen fibers have been shown to traverse the Golgi zone of chondrocytes before being released into the matrix.[28]

These studies indicate that in their route of synthesis, certain glycoprotein-containing substances such as mucus, secretory enzymes, and complex carbohydrates pass through the Golgi complex. All these cell products contain a significant amount of protein combined with carbohydrate. They are also substances destined to be secreted by the cells. Very recently it has been noted that proteins destined to be secreted, in contrast to those which are not secreted, are glycoproteins.[23] Although it is not known what role the carbohydrate serves, it may facilitate the release of secretory proteins from the cell.[23]

The Golgi complex is a major site for the synthesis of carbohydrate side chains which are to be linked to form mucopolysaccharides and glycoproteins. However, it does not appear to be the exclusive site for the manufacture of these side chains. Radioautographic studies of the formation of a glycoprotein in thyroid gland cells indicate that labeled galactose is incorporated in the Golgi complex but labeled mannose is taken up close to the ribosomes, where the protein portion of the molecule is formed.[23] Molecular analysis of this thyroid glycoprotein indicates that mannose units are located close to the protein, while galactose occurs nearer the ends of the side chains.[23] This has been taken as evidence that individual carbohydrate units are added in a stepwise sequence to the side chains of the glycoprotein. Presumably side-chain formation begins soon after the protein moiety is synthesized, mannose being added early and galactose later as the substance traverses the Golgi complex.[23]

Although the Golgi apparatus is a major synthesis site for some complex carbohydrates, [2,26] it does not appear to play the primary role in the synthesis of all these substances. For example, the complex carbohydrate *chondromucoprotein* is a major component of cartilage. Experimental evidence indicates that this particular substance is synthesized in the rough-surfaced and smooth-surfaced endoplasmic reticulum of chondrocytes, rather than in the Golgi apparatus.[11] It may, however, be concentrated in the Golgi region of the cell.

In certain cells, proteins may follow more than one pathway and not always traverse the Golgi apparatus before being released from the cell. Fibroblast cells of connective tissue provide an example. These cells produce large amounts of the fibrous extracellular protein *collagen*. It is thought that the fibroblasts synthesize tropocollagen molecules, which are precursors of the collagen fibril. The tropocollagen molecules are transported out of the cells and into the extracellular matrix. There, under the proper conditions, they associate themselves in such a way as to form collagen fibrils having a characteristic periodic pattern of cross striations every 700 Ångström units (Fig. V–14). In studies of collagen formation in wound healing, an intracellular accumulation of a secretory product (or precursor) within the Golgi complex of fibroblasts has not been observed.[30] It would appear that in this case tropocollagen may be secreted directly from the rough-surfaced endoplasmic reticulum into the extracellular space.[30]

It is already evident, from the few examples presented in this chapter, that cell organelles must function somewhat differently depending upon the specific products manufactured by the differentiated cell. That specialized cells are much alike in the organelles they contain is remarkable when one considers the variety of their products.

The following examples reemphasize the different kinds of substances manufactured: (1) The hormone *thyroxin* is synthesized by follicular cells of the thyroid gland. These cells release thyroxin into nearby capillaries so that via the blood stream the hormone reaches and exerts its effect upon various "target organs," thereby influencing the metabolism of the body. (2) The pancreas makes several compounds. Some are released directly into the blood (endocrine secretion) and others are released into a duct (exocrine secretion) which ultimately leads into the small intestine. The endocrine portions of the pancreas are called the Islets of Langerhans. Here, the two polypeptide hormones *insulin* and *glucagon* are manufactured and released into circulation. The largest portion of the pancreas, however, is concerned with the manufacture of enzymes that function in digestion. As we have discussed, these enzymes serve as a model for the synthesis and release of proteins. (3) *Steroids* are synthesized by certain cells in the adrenal cortex. Some of these steroid hormones play crucial roles in regulating the mineral metabolism of the body (for example, the retention or loss of potassium and sodium). At the present time we know only how a few substances are manufactured by cells. The cellular synthetic pathways of many other products remain to be elucidated.

REFERENCES

[1] Giuseppe Attardi, "The Mechanism of Protein Synthesis," *Ann. Rev. Microbiol.*, 21 (1967), 383–416.

[2] H. W. Beams and R. G. Kessel, "The Golgi Apparatus: Structure and Function," in *Intern. Rev. Cytol.*, G. H. Bourne and J. F. Danielli, eds. (New York: Academic Press Inc., 1968), Vol. 23, 209–276.

[3] H. S. Bennett, "Morphological Aspects of Extracellular Polysaccharides,"*J. Histochem. Cytocheml*, 11 (1963), 14–23.

[4] Bengt Borgström, "Absorption of Triglycerides," in *Lipid Transport*, H. C. Meng, ed. (Springfield, Ill., Charles C Thomas, 1964), 15–21.

[5] M. R. Capecchi, "Polypeptide Chain Termination *in Vitro:* Isolation of a Release Factor," *Proc. Nat. Acad. Sci.*, 58 (1967), 1144–1151.

[6] R. R. Cardell, Jr., Susan Badenhausen, and K. R. Porter, "Intestinal Triglyceride Absorption in the Rat. An Electron Microscopical Study," *J. Cell Biol.*, 34 (1967), 123–155.

[7] L. G. Caro and G. E. Palade, "Protein Synthesis, Storage, and Discharge in the Pancreatic Exocrine Cell," *J. Cell Biol.*, 20 (1964), 473–495.

[8] B. F. C. Clark and K. A. Marcker, "How Proteins Start," *Sci. Amer.*, 218 (1968), 36–42.

[9] F. H. C. Crick, "Nucleic Acids," *Sci. Amer.*, 197 (1957), 188–200.

[10] Henry Harris, *Nucleus and Cytoplasm* (New York: Oxford University Press, Inc., 1968).

[11] A. L. Horwitz and Albert Dorfman, "Subcellular Sites for Synthesis of Chondromucoprotein of Cartilage," *J. Cell Biol.*, 38 (1968), 358–368.

[12] Atsushi Ichikawa, "Fine Structural Changes in Response to Hormonal Stimulation of the Perfused Canine Pancreas," *J. Cell Biol.*, 24 (1965), 369–385.

[13] Susumu Ito, "Structure and Function of the Glycocalyx," *Fed. Proc.*, 28 (1969), 12–25.

[14] J. D. Jamieson and G. E. Palade, "Intracellular Transport of Secretory Proteins in the Pancreatic Exocrine Cell. I. Role of the Peripheral Elements of the Golgi Complex," *J. Cell Biol.*, 34 (1967), 577–596.

[15] J. D. Jamieson and G. E. Palade, "Intracellular Transport of Secretory Proteins in the Pancreatic Exocrine Cell. II. Transport to Condensing Vacuoles and Zymogen Granules," *J. Cell Biol.*, 34 (1967), 597–615.

[16] J. D. Jamieson and G. E. Palade, "Intracellular Transport of Secretory Proteins in the Pancreatic Exocrine Cell. III. Dissociation of Intracellular Transport from Protein Synthesis," *J. Cell Biol.*, 39 (1968), 580–588.

[17] J. D. Jamieson and G. E. Palade, "Intracellular Transport of Secretory Proteins in the Pancreatic Exocrine Cell. IV. Metabolic Requirements," *J. Cell Biol.*, 39 (1968), 589–603.

[18] J. M. Johnston and Bengt Borgström, "The Intestinal Absorption and Metabolism of Micellar Solutions of Lipids," *Biochim. Biophys. Acta*, 84 (1964), 412–423.

[19] A. L. Jones, N. B. Ruderman, and M. G. Herrera, "Electron Microscopic and Biochemical Study of Lipoprotein Synthesis in the Isolated Perfused Rat Liver," *J. Lipid Res.,* 8 (1967), 429–446.

[20] Hideko Kaji, Iwao Suzuka, and Akira Kaji, "Binding of Specific sRNA to Template Ribosome Complex: Effect of Proteolytic Enzymes," *J. Mol. Biol.,* 18 (1966), 219–234.

[21] Marian Neutra and C. P. Leblond, "Synthesis of the Carbohydrate of Mucus in the Golgi Complex as shown by Electron Microscope Radioautography of Goblet Cells from Rats Injected with Glucose-H³," *J. Cell Biol.,* 30 (1966), 119–136.

[22] Marian Neutra and C. P. Leblond, "Radioautographic Comparison of the Uptake of Galactose-H³ and Glucose-H³ in the Golgi Region of Various Cells Secreting Glycoproteins or Mucopolysaccharides," *J. Cell Biol.,* 30 (1966), 137–150.

[23] Marian Neutra and C. P. Leblond, "The Golgi Apparatus," *Sci. Amer.,* 220 (1969), 100–107.

[24] S. L. Palay and L. J. Karlin, "An Electron Microscopic Study of the Intestinal Villus. II. The Pathway of Fat Absorption," *J. Biophys. Biochem. Cytol.,* 5 (1959), 373–384.

[25] S. L. Palay and J.-P. Revel, "The Morphology of Fat Absorption," in *Lipid Transport,* H. C. Meng, ed. (Springfield, Ill., Charles C Thomas, 1964), 33–43.

[26] Marian Peterson and C. P. Leblond, "Synthesis of Complex Carbohydrates in the Golgi Region, as Shown by Radioautography after Injection of Labelled Glucose," *J. Cell Biol.,* 21 (1964), 143–148.

[27] C. M. Redman, P. Siekevitz, and G. E. Palade, "Synthesis and Transfer of Amylase in Pigeon Pancreatic Microsomes," *J. Biol. Chem.,* 241 (1966), 1150–1158.

[28] J.-P. Revel and E. D. Hay, "An Autoradiographic and Electron Microscopic Study of Collagen Synthesis in Differentiating Cartilage," *Z. Zellforsch.,* 61 (1963), 110–144.

[29] Alexander Rich, "The Structural Basis of Protein Synthesis," in *Molecular Organization and Biological Function,* John M. Allen, ed. (New York: Harper & Row, Inc., 1967), 20–36.

[30] Russell Ross and E. P. Benditt, "Wound Healing and Collagen Formation. V. Quantitative Electron Microscope Radioautographic Observations of Proline-H³ Utilization by Fibroblasts," *J. Cell Biol.,* 27 (1965), 83–106.

[31] D. Sabatini and Y. Tashiro, "Ribosomal Site of Attachment of Guinea Pig Liver Ribosomes to Microsomal Membranes," *Abstr. 6th Intern. Congr. Biochem. N.Y. I.U.B.,* 32 (1964), 84.

[32] Olga Stein and Yechezkiel Stein, "Fine Structure of the Ethanol Induced Fatty Liver in the Rat," *Israel J. Med. Sci.,* 1 (1965), 378–388.

[33] Mituru Takanami and Toshio Okamoto, "Interaction of Ribosomes and Synthetic Polyribonucleotides," *J. Mol. Biol.,* 7 (1963), 323–333.

VI

INTRA-CELLULAR DIGESTIVE TRACT:

Phagosome–Lysosome System

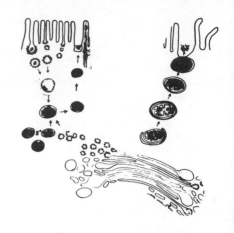

Various organelles in a cell work together to accomplish cell functions. For example, elements of the cell surface, the endoplasmic reticulum, the Golgi apparatus, and the lysosomes work in concert forming the intracellular digestive tract. Although the intracellular digestive tract may have developed to serve as a food-gathering function in unicellular organisms, the basic components of it have been modified during evolution to subserve a variety of complex and diverse functions in the multicellular organism. Some of these diverse functions are discussed in this chapter.

The intracellular digestive tract (or the phagosome–lysosome system) has components specialized for the following processes: (1) uptake of food substances within membrane-limited cavities; (2) the transfer of these substances within the cell; (3) their fusion with membrane-bound structures containing digestive enzymes; (4) the actual process of chemical digestion; and (5) the excretion or storage of waste materials. There are organelles associated with this phagosome–lysosome system which produce the digestive enzymes for its interior in a manner similar to that of the exocrine pancreas, which produces enzymes for the gastrointestinal tract. The cell accomplishes all these functions and yet protects itself from the potentially harmful digestive enzymes by conducting these processes within a membrane-limited space. Because of this compartmentalization, the digestive enzymes do not exist free in the cytoplasm. This membrane-limited space is at least potentially continuous with the extracellular space from which material is taken up and to which the residue is sometimes released.

Many investigators have contributed to our present understanding of the function of the intracellular digestive system. One particular scientist and his collaborators have played an extremely important role. De Duve and his associates, in addition to having discovered the presence of the organelle which contains the digestive (hydrolytic) enzymes, have provided much information of critical importance relating to various aspects of the system (see the excellent review of de Duve and Wattiaux).[9]

UPTAKE OF MATERIAL BY CELLS: ENDOCYTOSIS

It has long been known that certain cells have the ability to take up foreign material. *Phagocytosis,* or eating by cells, was described by Metchnikoff.[19] He discussed the nutritive function of phagocytosis in unicellular organisms and also stressed the importance of phagocytic cells in providing immunity for multicellular organisms.

Pinocytosis, or drinking by cells, was defined by Lewis.[16] He noted that certain cells in culture, such as macrophages, took up globules of fluid from the surrounding medium. These globules appeared within wavy veil-like pseudopodia near the cell periphery. The globules seemed to get caught up in the ruffle-like folds which formed around them. The globules then moved into the granular zone in the more central regions of the cell. Once there, they rapidly decreased in size until they became indistinguishable from other granules which were present in this zone. The term pinocytosis proposed by Lewis was applied by Mast and Doyle in 1934 to the uptake of fluid droplets by amoebae.[17] Certain substances present in the media induced the formation of pinocytic invaginations in the amoebae. Although the end result of the process in amoebae was the uptake of a fluid droplet, the morphology of pinocytosis differed from that observed by Lewis in macrophages. The first step in pinocytosis of proteins and colloidal suspensions by the amoeba *Chaos chaos* appeared to be the attachment of the substance to the cell membrane.[6] The next step was the uptake process. This involved the formation of channels and the subsequent pinching off of vacuoles from the bases of the channels.

Other epithelial cells from organs such as kidney and intestine can also segregate colloidal materials, dyes, and other proteins within vacuoles or granules in the same manner.[27]

A third process called *micropinocytosis,* or drinking of small quantities by cells, was identified in early electron microscopical investigations of various tissue types. In this process, small droplets of medium were trapped within invaginations of the cell membrane and then internalized by vesicle formation. The contents of the vesicle were not seen free in the cytoplasm but always separated from the cytoplasm by a membrane formed from the invaginating cell surface. Micropinocytotic processes have since been described in a variety of cells including the proximal tubular cells of the renal nephron, amoebae, erythroblasts, mosquito egg cells, hepatic cells, and epithelial cells lining various regions of the gastrointestinal tract.[9]

Because basic similarities exist in these various processes by which material can be taken into the cell, the term *endocytosis* has been applied to all of them.[8]

THE DISCOVERY OF LYSOSOMES

Lysosomes were first identified in centrifuged fractions of disrupted rat liver cells. When these disrupted rat liver cells were homogenized and the homogenate was fractionated by centrifugation at increasing speeds, a pellet formed in the bottom of the test tube at each speed. Resuspending one of these pellets resulted in a fraction that contained a variety of hydrolytic enzymes which showed a pH optimum in the acid range and hence were called *acid hydrolases*.[10]

Because there appeared to be a restriction on the accessibility of the internal hydrolases to external substrates and the fraction behaved like an osmotic system, it was inferred that the enzymes were contained in a membrane-bound structure. It was also demonstrated that the enzymes were released simultaneously under certain circumstances such as treatment with hypotonic solutions. Enzymes capable of breaking down all major types of compounds have been demonstrated in lysosomes.[9] These enzymes include acid phosphatase, acid ribonuclease, acid deoxyribonuclease, and acid proteases. A digestive role for lysosomes was therefore inferred by the presence of these hydrolytic enzymes.

It was later shown by electron microscopy that the lysosome fractions prepared from rat liver contained many organelles which appeared identical to bodies seen in sections of liver cells. These bodies had previously been called peribiliary dense bodies.[21] By modifying the light microscope Gomori technique for acid phosphatase for electron microscopy, acid phosphatase activity was demonstrated in the peribiliary dense bodies. Similar sac-like structures surrounded by single unit membranes have been seen in most cell types. The morphology of these bodies varies markedly from cell to cell. In some cells they appear pale in electron micrographs, while in others they appear dense. They sometimes have a relatively homogeneous matrix or can contain a variety of materials. When the cytochemical technique for demonstrating acid phosphatase is applied to tissues, the matrix of most of these bodies stain in a positive manner. This type of data has led to the suggestion that an intracellular organelle which stains positively for acid phosphatase and is bound by a single unit membrane may be a lysosome (Fig. VI–1).[20] Techniques more recently developed for use in conjunction with electron microscopy have demonstrated the presence of other hydrolytic enzymes in these same bodies.

These enzyme-containing bodies have been divided into two groups: *primary lysosomes* and *secondary lysosomes*. The primary (or virgin) lysosomes are bags of hydrolytic enzymes which have not yet been involved in the digestion of substances within cells. The secondary lysosomes are bodies which contain hydrolytic enzymes and which are either presently involved in the digestion of material or have completed the digestion of material. When secondary lysosomes are involved in the digestion of material taken in by endocytosis, they are referred to as heterophagic lysosomes. When the secondary lysosomes are involved in the digestion of material from within the cell, they are referred to as autophagic lysosomes.

LINKING OF ENDOCYTOSIS WITH LYSOSOMES

An unsuspected relationship between endocytosis and lysosomes was first recognized by Werner Straus in an important series of experiments involving protein uptake in the proximal convoluted tubular cells of the mammalian nephron.[26,28] When small proteins such as horseradish peroxidase are injected intravenously into animals, the protein is filtered through the renal corpuscle and gains access to the lumen of the connected nephron. The first part of the nephron is lined by proximal tubular cells. These cells normally reabsorb protein from the tubular lumen. In the Straus experiments, protein was injected into an animal, its kidney cells broken open and fractionated, and a purified particulate fraction prepared. It was found that the injected foreign protein and five lysosomal acid hydrolases existed together in that particular fraction.[26] In later studies, the enzyme protein horseradish peroxidase was again injected into animals. The cells of the proximal tubule took up the protein. In order to study the way in which these kidney cells handled the protein, the tissue was treated with a benzidine-containing solution to color the injected protein at various time intervals after protein administration. The same sections were treated to localize acid phosphatase activity. From these experiments[28] it was shown that injected protein first appeared in apical cytoplasmic droplets which did not stain histochemically for acid phosphatase. These were termed *phagosomes*. The phagosomes were formed by the process of endocytosis. At a later time, the phagosomes appeared to merge with acid phosphatase-positive lysosomes. After fusion the resulting bodies stained positively for both horseradish peroxidase and acid phosphatase. At later time intervals, the staining for horseradish peroxidase disappeared and only the acid phosphatase activity remained.

It was assumed that the loss of staining corresponded with the digestion of the horseradish peroxidase. It appears that other endogenous and exogenous proteins are handled in a similar manner.

The morphological details of this same process have been further clarified by the viewing of thin sections of tissue in an electron microscope.[14] First, the protein was filtered in the renal corpuscle (Fig. VI–2) and thereby gained access to the lumen of the proximal tubule. It then appeared to become concentrated inside the tubular invaginations which formed at the bases of the microvilli of these cells (Fig. VI–3). Small vesicles pinched off the invaginations and the protein was carried to larger vacuoles which were probably synonomous with the phagosomes seen in the light microscope (Fig. VI–4). The vacuoles became condensed and gained acid hydrolase activity presumably by fusing with primary or secondary lysosomes. These resulting peroxidase-containing granules had the morphological features of lysosomes (Fig. VI–5).

A similar endocytotic complex of invaginations, vesicles, and vacuoles has since been identified in many cell types and linked to protein sequestration and digestion.[13,15] A universal linking of the phagosome–lysosome system is evident from investigations of other cell systems. For example, studies with white blood cells (polymorphonuclear leucocytes) demonstrated a relationship between the uptake of bacteria into large vacuoles and the release of cytoplasmic granules (some of which were lysosomes) into these vacuoles.[7]

It therefore appeared that a variety of substances including proteins, bacteria, and debris could be taken up in various cell types by the formation of membrane-bound cavities. These cavities gained hydrolytic enzymes by fusing with primary or secondary lysosomes, and the contained material then underwent digestion. The products of digestion were thought to be small molecules which could pass through the lysosomal membrane. In general, these hydrolytic products are just beginning to be characterized. The specific hydrolases present within lysosomes and the end products produced by their activity may differ in various cell types.

It appears, however, that all substances are not completely degraded. Undigested residues of material such as ferritin and certain lipids remain in some lysosomes. The alteration of these lipid residues within lysosomes and the merging of these residual lysosomes are thought to lead to the formation of *lipofuscin pigment*, which is seen in certain cells during aging.[9] Protozoa eliminate debris from late food vacuoles by releasing it at the cell surface. In multicellular organisms, certain cells which border a lumen, such as the proximal tubular cells of the nephron and liver parenchymal cells, have been observed to release the debris contained within their residual lysosomes (Fig. VI–6).[24] This process involves the fusion of the lysosomal membrane with the cell surface membrane and the subsequent expulsion of the contents into the lumen.

AUTOPHAGIC VACUOLES

Living cells possess a mechanism by which they can segregate portions of their own cytoplasm for subsequent digestion. During this process, an area of cytoplasm becomes surrounded by a double-layered membranous sac. In what is presumed to be a later stage in the formation of the autophagic vacuole, one of the two membranes disappears, leaving a vacuole limited by a single membrane which contains morphologically recognizable cytoplasmic components in various stages of degradation (Fig. VI–7). That autophagic vacuoles are lysosomes is inferred from the observation that the autophagic vacuoles stain in a positive manner for acid phosphatase.

Autophagic vacuoles are present in many normal cells. They increase in number during certain normal processes such as differentiation, metamorphosis, hormonally induced changes in tissues, and aging. They are also more numerous in atrophy and in certain conditions of metabolic stress such as starvation. Autophagic vacuoles also form in sublethal reactions to a variety of injurious stimuli such as anoxia, excesses of certain hormones, or the administration of toxic compounds.[2,9]

The formation of autophagic vacuoles may also be the mechanism involved in organelle turnover within cells. It has been demonstrated that liver mitochondria are destroyed and renewed as a unit with a half-life on the order of 10.3 days.[12] It is unknown if organelles to be digested are selected at random or whether there is a means to discriminate which organelles need to be replaced.

A controversy has existed about the origin of the membranes which form around these portions of cytoplasm. Studies of autophagic vacuole formation in liver, after administration of the hormone glucagon,[2] showed that synthesis was not required to form the new membranes which limited autophagic vacuoles. By using enzymatic markers characteristic of various cell membranes, it was shown that the sac, which surrounded the cytoplasmic area to be digested, possessed the enzyme markers of the endoplasmic reticulum but not those of the Golgi apparatus, plasma membrane, or preexisting lysosomes.[2]

As the enclosed cellular organelles are digested they lose their distinguishing features, so that one cannot distinguish whether a given lysosome resulted from autophagic or heterophagic processes, or a combination of the two.

FORMATION OF PRIMARY LYSOSOMES BY CELLS

Primary lysosomes are lysosomes which have not yet been involved in digestion of material. Several hypotheses have been advanced to explain how primary lysosomes are formed within cells. It appears that the exact mechanism of primary lysosome formation may differ in various cell types. It is also conceivable that more than one pathway may operate in any given cell type.

Golgi Vesicles May Be Primary Lysosomes. One hypothesis concerning the formation of primary lysosomes proposes that they are formed in a manner similar to that used in the formation of digestive enzymes in exocrine pancreas cells (see Chapter V). The proteins appear to be manufactured by the ribosomes attached to the rough-surfaced endoplasmic reticulum. They are then apparently transferred to the Golgi apparatus by smooth-surfaced extensions of the endoplasmic reticulum. Subsequently they are released from the Golgi apparatus in vesicles, which are thought to be mature primary lysosomes.[20] This hypothesis is supported by the fact that acid phosphatase activity can be seen cytochemically in electron micrographs of Golgi cisternae and in Golgi vesicles.

A cell type which has been shown to utilize Golgi vesicles as primary lysosomes is that of the lining epithelium from vas deferens.[13] During protein uptake, a distinct population of small coated vesicles containing hydrolytic enzymes was derived from the Golgi complex. Some of these vesicles appeared to function in the transport of hydrolytic enzymes from the Golgi complex to the sites where digestion occurred.

Dense Granules May Be Primary Lysosomes. In certain cells, such as polymorphonuclear leucocytes, dense granules large enough to be seen in the light microscope appear to be primary lysosomes. These white blood cells are characterized by the presence of three distinct populations of granules.[3] The first population, called *azurophil granules,* has been shown to contain approximately 50 to 80 percent of the activity of five acid hydrolases, as well as myeloperoxidase activity, and one third of the activity of lysozyme (an antibacterial agent).[3] Because of this enzymatic activity, the azurophil granules can be considered to be primary lysosomes. These granules form early in the maturation of the cell from budding and subsequent aggregation of vacuoles on the concave surface of the Golgi apparatus.[4]

The GERL Hypothesis. The GERL hypothesis proposes that there is a region of the endoplasmic reticulum situated in the Golgi area which gives rise to lysosomal particles directly, in the form of both dense bodies and autophagic vacuoles.[8,22] The proponents of this hypothesis term this area the *GERL* (*G*olgi *E*ndoplasmic *R*eticulum *L*ysosomes). If this theory is correct, the hydrolytic enzymes do not necessarily traverse the Golgi apparatus, but, instead, this area of endoplasmic reticulum, which is associated both with the Golgi apparatus and the lysosomes, may be a site of intracellular digestive properties.

SPECIALIZED USES FOR THE PHAGOSOME–LYSOSOME SYSTEM

Although the phagosome–lysosome system may have originally evolved to serve a nutritive function in unicellular organisms, during the course of evolution it has been modified by cells to accomplish a diverse group of functions. The system plays an important role in host defense, bone resorption, and hormone secretion and regulation, as well as in fertilization, developmental processes, organelle turnover, and disposal or conservation of materials.[9]

Host Defense. Phagocytic cells of vertebrates use the phagosome–lysosome system to free the organism of foreign material. Polymorphonuclear leucocytes of the blood as well as a variety of mononuclear elements of the reticulo–endothelial system, such as macrophages, have the ability to engulf bacteria, cell debris, viruses, and toxic material.[7]

The polymorphonuclear leucocyte is an amoeboid cell which is produced in the bone marrow. It is then released into the vascular system, where it circulates for short periods of time. The cytoplasm of the cell contains several types of granules. The first population of granules is the azurophil granules, the primary lysosomes. The second population of granules, called *specific granules,* contains alkaline phosphatase and two thirds of the lysozyme. The third fraction is more heterogeneous; it also contains acid hydrolases but lacks peroxidase and lysozyme.[3] Under the appropriate stimulus, these polymorphonuclear leucocytes emigrate through vessel walls and are chemotactically attracted to areas that contain substances such as bacteria. The cells then engulf the invading bacteria and trap them in large invaginations. The invaginating membrane generally pinches off the cell surface leaving the bacteria in a membrane-bound vacuole. The leucocyte granules discharge their enzymatic contents into the phagocytic vacuole that surrounds the engulfed bacteria. This is accomplished by fusion of the vacuolar membrane with that surrounding the granule (Fig. VI–8). These lytic enzymes presumably attack and digest the bacteria while the cell remains in good health.[7]

The Secretion of Lysosomal Enzymes for Extracellular Use. It appears that, in special circumstances, lysosomes secrete their enzymes into the extracellular space so that the enzymes may act outside the cell. This phenomenon occurs during the resorption of bone by osteoclasts.[29] Bone resorption in tissue culture is accompanied by the release of six lysosomal acid hydrolases but not by a release of the nonlysosomal enzymes measured. It appears that the lysosomal enzymes are released by fusion of the membrane surrounding the lysosome with the surface membrane in a manner similar to the release of lysosomal enzymes into digestive vacuoles. The acid hydrolases appear to be active in the resorption of the organic matrix of the bone.

Role in Hormone Release. The thyroid is an endocrine gland which produces thyroid hormones. It is composed of follicles which consist of a lumen filled with colloid surrounded by a single layer of cells. Cells from the thyroid follicle, when stimulated with *thyrotropic hormone* (TSH), exhibit morphologic evidence of active uptake of colloid by endocytosis.[23] At first, the newly formed colloid droplets lack acid phosphatase activity. However, at later time periods the droplets are positive for acid phosphatase. Apparently the colloid droplets fuse with dense lysosome-like bodies.

Thyroglobin is the hormone precursor in the colloid droplets. Before being released from the cell, the thyroid hormones are split from the globulin. The splitting of the thyroid hormones from thyroglobulin is the proposed function of the hydrolytic enzymes.[23] However, if this is the case, the enzymes present in thyroid lysosomes must differ from those found in lysosomes of other better-studied cells because hydrolytic breakdown in thyroid lysosomes apparently leaves the thyroid hormones intact.

Hormone Regulation by Lysosomes. It has been postulated that lysosomes play a role in segregation and degradation of protein produced by the cell.[25] Evidence for such a theory is based upon experimental data from the *mammotrophic hormone* (MTH or LTH), produced by the cells of the rat pituitary gland, and appearing in the cytoplasm as granules. The amount of hormone secreted was high during lactation and was low after removal of the young. During periods of high hormone production, the cells were characterized by the presence of well-developed protein-synthesizing apparatus and forming secretory granules. After the young were removed, the lysosomes were seen to incorporate and degrade the excess secretory granules. Concomitant with this, areas of endoplasmic reticulum and ribosomes were sequestered into autophagic vacuoles for digestion.

This experiment indicates that lysosomes function in the regulation of secretory processes by the digestion of excess granules.

THE ROLE OF THE PHAGOSOME–LYSOSOME SYSTEM IN DISEASE

The participation of the phagosome–lysosome system in certain pathologic conditions has been suggested.[31] *Pompe's disease* (or glycogen storage disease type II) is a type of specific lysosomal disease.[5] It appears to result from a congenital absence of one lysosomal hydrolytic enzyme called α-glucosidase. The enzyme normally functions in the degradation of glycogen and its lack results in a deposition of unmetabolized substrate (in this case, glycogen) in liver lysosomes.[5]

Another disease, *metachromatic leukodystrophy,* results in the accumulation of sulphated mucopolysaccharide in nervous tissue. This process has been associated with a defect in the lysosomal enzyme aryl sulfatase A.[1,18]

It is likely that certain other diseases result from similar defects in lysosomal hydrolases.[31] One interesting aspect in diseases of this type is that these deficient lysosomes may be accessible to replacement therapy. It is possible that administration of the missing lysosomal enzyme to a patient could result in enzyme uptake by the phagsome–lysosome system with subsequent digestion of the excess substrate within the lysosomes.

Fragility of lysosomes in tissues may also cause injury and disease. Circumstantial evidence exists which links rheumatoid arthritis to lysosomal fragility. The erosion of the cartilage matrix which occurs in this disease appears to be related to the release of lysosomal enzymes by the invading cells.[11] Agents which can rupture lysosomes (so-called labilizers) tend to aggravate rheumatoid arthritis, while substances which promote lysosomal stability, such as chloroquine and cortisone, tend to ameliorate rheumatic diseases.[30]

REFERENCES

[1]James Austin, Donald McAfee, Donald Armstrong, Michael O'Rourke, Leslie Shearer, and Bismal Bachhawat, "Abnormal Sulphatase Activities in Two Human Diseases (Metachromatic Leucodystrophy and Gargoylism)," *Biochem. J.,* 93 (1964) 15c–17c.

[2]A. U. Arstila and B. F. Trump, "Studies on Cellular Autophagocytosis. The Formation of Autophagic Vacuoles in the Liver after Glucagon Administration," *Amer. J. Path.,* 53 (1968), 687–733.

[3]Marco Baggiolini, J. G. Hirsch, and Christian de Duve, "Resolution of Granules from Rabbit Heterophil Leukocytes into Distinct Populations by Zonal Sedimentation," *J. Cell Biol.,* 40 (1969), 529–541.

[4]D. F. Bainton and M. G. Farquhar, "Origin of Granules in Polymorphonuclear Leukocytes," *J. Cell Biol.,* 28 (1966), 277–301.

[5]P. Baudhuin, H. G. Hers, and H. Loeb, "An Electron Microscopic and Biochemical Study of Type II Glycogenosis," *Lab. Invest.,* 13 (1964), 1139–1152.

[6]P. W. Brandt and G. D. Pappas, "An Electron Microscopic Study of Pinocytosis in Amoeba. I. The Surface Attachment Phase," *J. Biophys. Biochem. Cytol.,* 8 (1960), 675–687.

[7]Z. A. Cohn, J. G. Hirsch, and Edith Wiener, "The Cytoplasmic Granules of Phagocytic Cells and the Degradation of Bacteria," in *Lysosomes,* A. V. S. de Reuck and M. P. Cameron, eds., Ciba Found., Gen. Symp. (Boston, Little, Brown and Co., 1963), 126–150.

[8]Christian de Duve, "The Lysosome Concept," in *Lysosomes,* A. V. S. de Reuck and M. P. Cameron, eds., Ciba Found., Gen. Symp. (Boston: Little, Brown and Co., 1963), 1–35.

[9]Christian de Duve and Robert Wattiaux, "Functions of Lysosomes," *Ann. Rev. Physiol.,* 28 (1966), 435–492.

[10]Christian de Duve, B. C. Pressman, R. Gianetto, Robert Wattiaux, and F. Appelmans, "Tissue Fractionation Studies. 6. Intracellular Distribution Patterns of Enzymes in Rat-Liver Tissue," *Biochem. J.,* 60 (1955), 604–617.

[11]J. T. Dingle, "Aetiological Factors in the Collagen Diseases: Lysosomal Enzymes and the Degradation of Cartilage Matrix," *Proc. Royal Soc. Med.* (London), 55 (1962), 109–111.

[12]M. J. Fletcher and D. R. Sanadi, "Turnover of Rat-Liver Mitochondria," *Biochem. Biophys. Acta,* 51 (1961), 356–360.

[13]D. S. Friend and M. G. Farquhar, "Functions of Coated Vesicles during Protein Absorption in the Rat Vas Deferens," *J. Cell Biol.,* 35 (1967), 357–376.

[14]R. C. Graham, Jr., and M. J. Karnovsky, "The Early Stages of Absorption of Injected Horseradish Peroxidase in the Proximal Tubules of Mouse Kidney: Ultrastructural Cytochemistry by New Technique," *J. Histochem. Cytochem.,* 14 (1966), 291–302.

[15]D. O. Graney, "The Uptake of Ferritin by Ileal Absorptive Cells in Suckling Rats. An Electron Microscope Study," *Amer. J. Anat.,* 123 (1968), 227–254.

[16]W. H. Lewis, "Pinocytosis," *Bull. Johns Hopkins Hosp.,* 49 (1931), 17–27.

[17]S. O. Mast and W. L. Doyle, "Ingestion of Fluid by Amoeba," *Protoplasma,* 20 (1934), 555–560.

[18]Ehrenfried Mehl and Horst Jatzkewitz, "Über ein Cerebrosidschwefelsäureester spaltendes Enzym aus Schweineniere," *Hoppe-Seyler's Z. Physiol. Chem.,* 331 (1963), 292–294.

[19]Elie Metchnikoff, *Immunity in Infective Diseases* (Cambridge, University Press, 1905).

[20]A. B. Novikoff, "Lysosomes in the Physiology and Pathology of Cells: Contributions of Staining Methods," in *Lysosomes,* A. V. S. de Reuck and M. P. Cameron, eds., Ciba Found., Gen . Symp. (Boston: Little, Brown and Co., 1963), 36–77.

[21]A. B. Novikoff, H. Beufay, and Christian de Duve, "Electron Microscopy of Lysosome-Rich Fractions from Rat Liver," *J. Biophys. Biochem. Cytol.,* 2, No. 4, Suppl. (1956), 179–184.

[22]A. B. Novikoff, Nelson Quintana, Humberto Villaverde, and Regina Forschirm, "The Golgi Zone of Neurons in Rat Spinal Ganglia," *J. Cell Biol.,* 23 (1964), 68A.

[23]Rolf Seljelid, "Endocytosis in Thyroid Follicle Cells. IV. On the Acid Phosphatase Activity in Thyroid Follicle Cells with Special Reference to the Quantitative Aspects," *J. Ultrastruct. Res.,* 18 (1967), 237–256.

[24]T. K. Shnitka, "Pinocytotic Labelling of Liver-Cell Lysosomes with Colloidal Gold: Observations of the Uptake of the Marker, and its Subsequent Discharge into Bile Canaliculi," *Fed. Proc.,* 24 (1965), 556.

[25]R. E. Smith and M. G. Farquhar, "Lysosome Function in the Regulation of the Secretory Process in Cells of the Anterior Pituitary Gland," *J. Cell Biol.,* 31 (1966), 319–347.

[26]Werner Straus, "Concentration of Acid Phosphatase, Ribonuclease, Desoxyribonuclease β-Glucuronidase, and Cathepsin in 'Droplets' Isolated from the Kidney Cells of Normal Rats," *J. Biophys. Biochem. Cytol.,* 2 (1956), 513–521.

[27]Werner Straus, "Comparative Observations on Lysosomes and Phagosomes in Kidney and Liver of Rats after Administration of Horseradish Peroxidase," in *Lysosomes,* A. V. S. de Reuck and M. P. Cameron, eds., Ciba Found., Gen. Symp. (Boston, Little, Brown and Co., 1963), 151–175.

[28]Werner Straus, "Changes in Intracellular Location of Small Phagosomes (Micropinocytic Vesicles) in Kidney and Liver Cells in Relation to Time after Injection and Dose of Horseradish Peroxidase," *J. Histochem. Cytochem.,* 15 (1967), 381–393.

[29]Gilbert Vaes, "On the Mechanisms of Bone Resorption," *J. Cell Biol.,* 39 (1968), 676–697.

[30]Gerald Weissmann, "Labilization and Stabilization of Lysosomes," *Fed. Proc.,* 23 (1964), 1038–1044.

[31]Gerald Weissmann, "Lysosomes," *New Eng. J. Med.,* 273 (1965), 1084–1090, 1143–1149.

VII

THE SPECIALIZED CELL

CELL DIFFERENTIATION

The development of a single cell (the fertilized egg) into the many specialized cells comprising the tissues of a multicellular animal is one of the most intriguing subjects in biology. The progress of cells toward increased specialization in structure and function is known as differentiation. Differentiation is the basis of development and, as its consequence, various parts of an organism become restricted and acquire the ability to perform special functions.[9] For example, heart muscle cells are highly specialized to beat rhythmically and continuously throughout life. Melanocytes in the skin are differentiated to produce melanin pigment granules in their cytoplasm. These granules in turn function as a barrier to filter out harmful and excessive rays of sunlight. These differentiated cells still carry out the normal metabolic processes necessary to maintain homeostasis, but, in addition, they are specialized to perform certain functions that other cells are incapable of performing. All these specialized cell types existing in a single animal developed from the same fertilized egg.

For a number of years it was thought that the cytoplasm was responsible for cell differentiation. This idea gained support because it was known that during mitotic cell division, identical sets of chromosomes, with their hereditary carriers the genes, passed to daughter cells. Because all the cells of an individual were genetically identical, it seemed unlikely that genes could be responsible for regulating the development of different, specialized cell types. Furthermore, it was noted that most cell specializations occurred in the absence of mitotic division. So again, any significant role that might be played by the nucleus was overlooked. The major factors influencing cell differentiation were ascribed to unequal cytoplasmic division and the changing external environment of the cell.

Some investigators began to feel uneasy about excluding the chromosomes from a role in cell specialization. It was then discovered that genetic mutations could block specific steps in the developmental process. In a review article published in 1961, Jacob and Monod[16] proposed a convincing theory that changed the thinking about the function of genes. They demonstrated that mutant strains of the bacterium *Escherichia coli* could be induced by lactose to synthesize the enzyme β-galactosidase. Originally the mutant bacterium had very low amounts of this enzyme. When lactose was added to the medium the bacterium began to synthesize β-galactosidase at a rapid rate. Soon its concentration within the bacterial cell was increased about 1,000 times. The Jacob and Monod theory postulated that the genes responsible for the production of β-galactosidase were *repressed* until lactose acted as an *inducer* to derepress these genes and permit them to function.[14] Additional studies with other organisms have shown that various molecules can act as signals (i.e., analogous to lactose in the example just cited) to bring inactive genes into states of functional activity.

In Chapter V we reviewed the two central parts of the concept of gene action: *transcription* and *translation*. The genetic information coded in the nucleotide base sequence of deoxyribonucleic acid (DNA) is *transcribed* into a complementary nucleotide base sequence in messenger ribonucleic acid (mRNA). The mRNA then temporarily unites with ribosomes where the nucleotide sequence of the mRNA is *translated* into the amino acid sequence of a particular protein. It is the synthesis of mRNA that appears to be regulated by various molecules.[16] The mRNA acts to specify the kinds of proteins synthesized, and the proteins to a large extent characterize a particular type of specialized cell. In general, mRNA usually has a short lifetime, and if no new mRNA directing a particular enzyme is being made, the ribosomal machinery for manufacture of that enzyme is disassembled within minutes or hours.

The concept that genes exist in *active and inactive states* gave important clues to what occurred in cell differentiation. Although all cells in the same animal have identical sets of genes, only certain genes are active at any one time in the process of development. The cytoplasm of cells differs in the kinds of product molecules they contain, depending upon which of the genes are functioning.

When does a cell become differentiated? Is it when a specialized protein first becomes biochemically detectable (for example, myosin in a muscle cell), or is it when discernible structures (for example, myofibrils) first make their appearance within the cytoplasm? At some point in time the fate of a cell becomes determined. Perhaps differentiation occurs sometime before obvious cytoplasmic differences are expressed. Generally, both biochemical and morphological criteria are used to detect the changes accompanying the specialization process. As differentiation occurs within cells, corresponding changes are also observed at the tissue level. These in turn are expressed at the organizational level of the whole embryo as it gradually attains its diverse organ systems.

Cell specialization, although under genetic control, requires the interaction of both the nucleus and the cytoplasm. We have already discussed (see Chapter IV) how one important aspect of cell specialization—the determination of cell shape—depends upon this interaction. The genes present within the nucleus of a cell and the substrates present within its cytoplasm determine the particular pathway of specialization. Changes in the nucleus are expressed in the cytoplasm, and, conversely, changes in the cytoplasm affect nuclear activity. Once differentiated, a cell is reasonably stable because the gene activation has produced altered nuclear–cytoplasmic interaction. A nerve cell remains a nerve cell and a kidney cell functions strictly as a kidney cell throughout its entire lifetime, which in some cases corresponds to the lifetime of the animal. In other cases (for example, in the production of blood cells), final differentiation occurs after cell division of a less differentiated *stem cell*. These fully differentiated cells have only a limited lifetime and must be renewed frequently. The mechanisms which regulate and control gene activity appear to be involved in the maintenance of the differentiated state.[4] Although much remains to be learned about the way genes are regulated, a few lines of evidence offer some insight into the problem.

Chromosome Puffs. The larval stages of certain insects have giant chromosomes in some of their cells. These *polytene chromosomes* consist of many hundreds of identical strands arranged in register parallel to one another. As a result of this ordered pattern, the chromosomes display a specific linear sequence of cross bands. At particular times during the development of the insect, a given position (crossband) along the chromosome changes from a band to a puff. The puffs appear as swollen thickenings and it appears as if the chromosomal thread has uncoiled at a given locus. It has been shown that in certain salivary gland cells of developing insects a particular puff is associated with the appearance of a distinct granular secretion and differentiation into a secretory cell type.[2] Not all the salivary gland cell chromosomes show this puff, but those that do begin to display evidence of the secretory product. Moreover, it has been discovered that some strains of insects fail to show this particular puff in the giant chromosomes of their salivary gland cells. These chromosomes maintain condensed bands at this site and the cells do not differentiate into secretory cells. As a result, these are "nonsecreting" strains of insects. Therefore, the puffs represent gene activity and this particular puff is correlated with differentiation into a secretory cell.

A molting hormone ecdysone has been shown to alter the puff pattern when administered to developing insects.[5] Presumably it directly or indirectly acts to derepress certain genes. The products of these activated genes (or perhaps the derepressed genes themselves) in turn derepress other genes in a sequential pattern. Varying the amount of a hormone and/or administering combinations of various hormones cause different puffing patterns. Hormones presumably do play important roles in regulating gene activity, but their exact mechanisms of action are unknown.

A significant factor in maintaining cell specialization seems to be the control of mRNA synthesis.[16] The lifetime of mRNAs varies from minutes in some bacteria to many hours or weeks in other oganisms. Differentiated cells apparently continue to produce certain kinds of mRNA which persist for long periods and which perhaps even replicate themselves. They in turn function to produce the specific kinds of proteins that characterize and stabilize the differentiated cell.

Bristle Formation in *Drosophila*. In studies with the fly *Drosophila* it has been shown that pattern is under genetic control.[25] These insects have a particular number and arrangement of bristles projecting through the chitinous armor that covers their body. Each bristle moves as if it were a joint, and is housed within a socket in the armor. The bristles are part of a complex sensory organ that consists of three differentiated cells (Fig. VII–1). All three of these specialized cells develop from one ancestral "bristle organ" cell. The original cell divides and one of its daughters forms the sensory nerve cell; the other daughter divides again and the two progeny form the bristle cell and the socket cell. The bristle cell secretes the bristle outgrowth, while the socket cell produces a substance which forms a ring to enclose the bristle shaft. Underlying these two cells is a short sensory nerve which leads from the bristle organ into the central nervous system.

Mutant strains of *Drosophila* (i.e., those carrying the gene "hairless") lack certain bristles and therefore are characterized by a pattern difference.[25] It has been shown that a mutation in the DNA of the ancestral

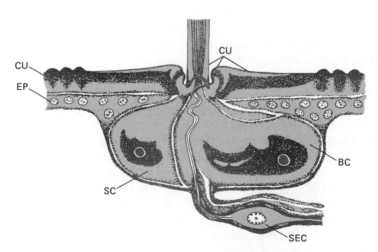

FIGURE VII–1. Bristle apparatus consisting of bristle cell (BC), socket cell (SC), and sensory cell (SEC), all embedded in the cuticule (CU) and epidermis (EP). Semidiagrammatic. Modified from Curt Stern, *Amer. Sci.,* 42 (1954), 213.

sense organ cell affects its ability to differentiate into a normal bristle organ. Instead, the two cells which usually differentiate into a bristle cell and a socket cell both differentiate into socket cells. The only explanation for this alteration is the presence of a "hairless" gene. Further support for the bristle being the end product of gene action was shown by experimental studies. There was an increase in the size of bristles in adult flies that developed from eggs which had been experimentally given two or three genes for bristle length. Moreover, genetically crossing various *Drosophila* (strains having bristles of different shapes and lengths) resulted in particular bristle shapes and patterns. These results clearly indicate that genetic control is responsible for the expressed alteration in bristle shape.

The Ciliate Cortex. The discovery of different states of gene activity shifted the focus of attention to the role played by the nucleus in cell differentiation. There are, however, some aspects of cell differentiation that cannot be accounted for by genetic activity and that appear to be independent of them. This is most impressively demonstrated by work with *Paramecium*, a ciliated protozoan.[24] This complex cell normally divides in half transversely and produces two identically structured cells (not two different cell halves as if the cell were merely cut in two). Individual *Paramecia* can be experimentally altered so that they have two or more mouth structures. When the altered cells divide, their progeny inherit the additional mouth structures. Nuclear transplantations between these and normal *Paramecia* do not affect the altered *Paramecia* and this cortical structure abnormality can be propagated for many successive divisions. In fact, for hundreds of cell generations, similar experimental alterations have been perpetuated. Preexisting cell structures somehow influence the location and arranging of new molecules (which the genes were originally responsible for producing). There is evidence in these *Paramecia* experiments that something other than the genes stores information and transmits it in the form of existing cortical patterns. Other scientists have stressed the importance of what is still to be learned about the factors which influence the development of animal cells.[13] Cytoplasmic factors may play a more significant role than is presently appreciated.

Mitochondrial DNA. In the early 1960s it was demonstrated that DNA was not located exclusively in the nucleus, but was also present in certain cytoplasmic organelles.[17] We mentioned in Chapter III that DNA (and RNA) are definite components of mitochondria and chloroplasts. Mitochondrial DNA usually exists as a circular double-stranded structure, in contrast to the characteristic double helix of nuclear DNA from multicellular animals. It has been shown that mitochondrial DNA can replicate itself. Mitochondria can also synthesize RNA (which is distinctly different from that of the cytoplasm), and incorporate amino acids into protein. A substantial amount of evidence favors a genetic role for mitochondrial

DNA. However, it appears that in order to code for all the components necessary to synthesize a mitochondrion, mitochondrial DNA is inadequate. Therefore, it is thought that the nuclear genetic system interacts with that of the mitochondrion in order to achieve organelle biosynthesis.[17]

It has long been recognized that mitochondrial morphology and function directly reflects the metabolic state of a cell. In certain pathological conditions alterations in mitochondria are clearly evident and the possibility arises that the structure of mitochondrial DNA might also be altered. In fact, altered mitochondrial DNA in mutant yeast cells has resulted in important inherited changes in the structure and function of their mitochondria.[17] This population of altered mitochondria was membrane deficient and lacked certain enzymes necessary for normal metabolism.

EXAMPLES OF SPECIALIZED CELLS

In order to emphasize the degree of specialization that can be attained by cells, selected examples of mammalian cell types are discussed. These include photoreceptor cells of the retina, and skeletal muscle cells.

Rod and Cone Cells: Photoreception. Rod and cone cells of the retina are among some of the most highly differentiated cells. They function to receive light and to transform it into nerve impulses that travel to the occipital cortex of the brain, where vision is experienced. Each specialized photoreceptor cell consists of two parts, an *outer segment* and an *inner segment,* connected to one another by a slender cytoplasmic process. The rod and cone cells are arranged with their protruding outer segments facing toward the back of the eye. Light, therefore, passes through most layers of the retina before reaching the light-sensitive portion of these cells. Photoreceptor cells are named by the shape of their outer segments. Those of rods are long slender cylinders, while those of cones are tapered into a conical shape. The photoreceptor cells differ in their sensitivity and response to light. Rod cells function in light of very low intensity and make night vision possible (the dark-adapted eye). Cone cells are less sensitive to light of low intensity, but are responsible for color vision.

When sectioned and examined in the electron microscope, the outer segments of both types of photoreceptor cells display many stacks of lamellar membranes arranged at an angle perpendicular to the long axis of the rod cell (Fig. VII–2). The lamellar membranes are flattened into sac-like discs (approximately 140 Ångström units thick) which contain light-sensitive pigments, *rhodopsin* in rods and *iodopsin* in cones. At the basal region of the outer segment and located at one side of the cell is a slender cytoplasmic connection, called a *stalk.* When cut in cross section, the stalk reveals the nine outer doublet microtubules characteristic of most cilia but the two central fibrils are lacking. Studies of developing rods indicate that their outer segments actually do arise from modified cilia. Their differentiation includes the following major steps:[7] the inner segment of a developing rod cell contains a pair of centrioles which are located at angles perpendicular to one another. From one of these centrioles a modified cilium emerges and pushes its way apically, forcing out a bulb of cytoplasm around it. "Morphogenetic material" consisting of tubular and membranous elements surrounds the cilium as it grows. The bulbous protrusion of cytoplasm surrounding the primitive cilium enlarges, and portions of the cell membrane begin to invaginate into it forming vesicular sacs. These sacs are at first disorganized, then they become oriented and remolded into the flattened lamellar discs characteristic of the fully developed outer segment. The discs pinch off the cell membrane but adjacent discs remain interconnected to one another.

The inner segment of the rod cell also displays morphological alterations during development. It contains most of the enzymes responsible for supplying energy to the cell. This segment of the rod has two distinct regions. The outermost part contains the basal body of the connecting cilium and is packed with mitochondria which function to supply energy. The inner portion lacks mitochondria but contains Golgi elements, endoplasmic reticulum, and fibrous elements. The fibrous elements organize themselves into a definite bundle. The remaining part of the cell constitutes the *rod fiber*. This portion of the rod cell is a slender protoplasmic process that has characteristics very similar to an unmyelinated nerve fiber. The rod cell nucleus is contained within this part of the cell. From the nucleus, the rod fiber elements continue deeper, to the most proximal end of the cell, where *synaptic contacts* are formed with bipolar nerve cells.

The *bipolar nerve cells* are part of the next-deeper retinal layer. Their unusual contacts with the rod photoreceptor cells are very important in transferring the generated signal of light reception to the nerve circuits that continue to the visual centers of the brain. In their areas of synaptic contact, these two cells exhibit a complex and intricate relationship.[23] The rod cell exhibits a bulbous swelling. Penetrating into deep invaginations on the internal aspect of this swelling are processes of the bipolar cell (somewhat analogous to fingers being pushed into a balloon). These dendritic bipolar cell processes make contact with two large vacuoles also located within the invagination of the rod cell membrane. Situated between the two large vacuoles in the rod cell is a structure called a *synaptic ribbon* (Fig. VII–3). The synaptic ribbon stains very intensely and appears as a rod or disc flanked by a number of small vesicles. Synaptic ribbons are associated with many sensory receptor cells. Their specific function remains unknown, but they must function in some way to transmit to the bipolar cell the electrical disturbance that is set up in the rod cell when light strikes it.

Exactly how the photoreceptor cell performs its function of receiving light and transforming it into nerve impulses is not completely understood. However, we do know some of the chemical events involved in the absorption of light by the rod outer segment. The pigment *rhodopsin* is contained within the lamellar discs of rod outer segments, while *iodopsin* exists in cone outer segments. These pigment molecules function to absorb quanta of light. Rhodopsin and iodopsin consist of vitamin A aldehyde *(retinene)*, conjugated to a specific protein (rod *opsin* or cone *opsin*).[3] The retinene portion of these pigment molecules can exist in any one of five isomeric forms. The biochemical processes associated with visual excitation are best understood with regard to the rhodopsin molecule. Retinene exists in unbleached rhodopsin as the 11-cis isomer. Exposure to visible light triggers a series of conformational changes within the rhodopsin molecule converting the isomer (through a series of short-lived intermediates) to the all-trans conformation. Following this series of biochemical reactions, there is apparently a depolarization of the rod cell membrane. An action potential is formed and propagated (across the cell gap) to the bipolar cell. Crossing several more synapses it then travels along the optic nerve tract to the brain.

Our present knowledge of what happens to link the biochemical reactions to the membrane depolarization is exceedingly scanty. In fact, despite claims that the rod cell membrane is depolarized, electrophysiologists have not yet been able to record an action potential from these photoreceptor cells. To explain the mechanism of visual excitation, a few hypothetical proposals have been made.[26] When light strikes a pigment molecule, it is conceivable that a hole is created in the lamellar disc membrane. This event may cause a depolarization that is propagated along the discs which are interconnected to one another. Another possibility is that rhodopsin, when activated by light, undergoes molecular rearrangement that unmasks certain chemical groupings. These newly exposed chemical sites could have an increased ability to bind ions and as a consequence the altered rhodopsin may act as an enzyme.[26] Chemical cycles of response and recovery could be initiated as the rhodopsin catalyzes the formation of many product molecules, and these chemical cycles could characterize the process of visual excitation. The events that follow this initial activation, and the detailed mechanism of synaptic transmission from the rod cell to the bipolar cell, remain unknown.

Skeletal Muscle Cells and Contraction. A striated muscle cell provides one of the best examples of a highly differentiated cell where a workable understanding of structure and function has been obtained (Fig. VII–4). When fresh skeletal muscle is experimentally teased apart, many long cylindrical multinucleated muscle cells are obtained. Under a dissecting microscope, these muscle cells exhibit longitudinal and cross striations. The striations are due to the repeating pattern of the components of

SKELETAL MUSCLE

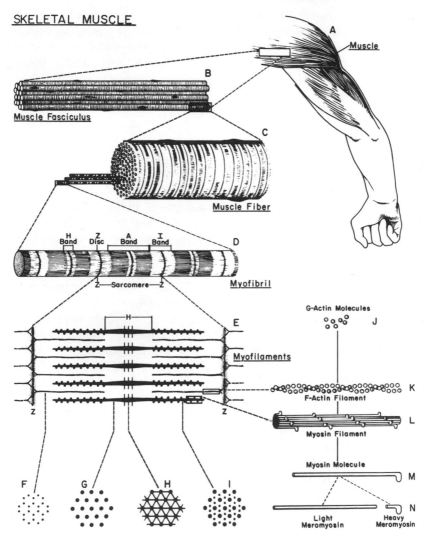

FIGURE VII–4. Diagram of the organization of skeletal muscle. Courtesy of W. Bloom and D. W. Fawcett, *A Textbook of Histology,* W. B. Saunders Co., Philadelphia, 1968.

the *myofibrils* within the cytoplasm of the muscle cell. Each myofibril is composed of bundles of *myofilaments* arranged parallel to one another and to the long axis of the muscle cell (Fig. VII–5). The myofilaments appear to play a significant role in muscle contraction. The fine structure of striated muscle cell myofibrils reveals characteristic banding patterns. A darkly stained *A* band (so named because it is *anisotropic* or *birefringent* when examined with polarized light) alternates with a light staining *I* band *(isotropic* or *singly refractile).* These two major bands are roughly the same length and within each of them additional bands are observed. The dark *A* band has a lighter central area designated as an *H* band, and in the center of the *H* band is a dark *M* band. The *I* band has a most obvious dark narrow *Z* band bisecting its center, and the unit of length between two such *Z* bands (about 2.5 microns in relaxed muscle) is called a *sarcomere* (Fig. VII–6).

Two kinds of fibrous proteins, *myosin* and *actin,* are the main constituents of myofilaments.[12,14] The thicker of the two filaments measures approximately 150 Ångström units in diameter and is primarily myosin. Actin forms the major part of the thinner filament that measures about 60 Ångström units in diameter. A myofibril cross-sectioned through the *A* band displays a very precise arrangement of these thick and thin filaments (Fig. VII–6 inset). Each myosin filament is seen surrounded by six thin filaments arranged in a hexagonal pattern. The two sets of filaments (actin and myosin) in the *A* band account for its birefringence (meaning that it has two different indexes of refraction). The thick myosin filaments are limited exclusively to the *A* band and are all the same length, being arranged in register parallel to one another (Fig. VII–4). The *A* band therefore measures the same as the length of a myosin filament, about 1.5 microns in frog or rabbit leg muscle. The thin filaments originate at the *Z* bands, run through the *I* band and into the *A* band between the thick filaments to end at the edge of the *H* band. These filaments measure about 1 micron in length and they also are arranged in register parallel to one another. Between adjacent thick and thin filaments, *cross bridges* are observed.[12,14] The cross bridges are part of the thick myosin filaments, a finding related to the observation that they are clearly evident in the *H* band, where only thick filaments are observed. The cross bridges are the only visible structural link between the two sets of filaments and they are thought to play an important role in the process of contraction.

Closely associated with the myofibrils within the muscle cell are mitochondria (which supply energy to the cell), and a complex system of internal membranes called the *sarcoplasmic reticulum.* This network is a modification of the smooth-surfaced endoplasmic reticulum (Figs. VII–5, VII–7) that is closely associated with the myofibrils. It extends around these filament bundles and bears a characteristic relationship to certain of their bands. The sac-like elements of the sarcoplasmic reticulum can be seen flanking a central tubule *(T-tubule* or transverse tubule) and forming the so-called *triads* of skeletal muscle (Fig. VII–7). The central *T*-tubule has been shown to be a deep invagination of the external cell membrane, making it separate from the internal membranes which constitute the sarcoplasmic reticulum.[20] (Figure VII–8 demonstrates the tracer horseradish peroxidase in these deep *T*-tubule invaginations, indicating their communication with the extracellular space.) From this discovery it became apparent that via the *T*-tubule extension a signal for contraction could quickly be conducted the rather long distance from the peripheral surface of the muscle cell membrane into the central area of the muscle cell.

An understanding of the relationship between contraction and these many structural specializations is being realized. Step by step the molecular events associated with contraction are being elucidated. In the light microscope, it was possible to observe changes in the banding pattern of striated muscle during contraction. The length of the *A* band remained constant, but the *H* band disappeared and the *I* band decreased in length. Because the fine structure of muscle was not known at that time, no good explanation of contraction was possible. The *sliding filament hypothesis* of muscle contraction proposed by Hugh Huxley and coworkers[12,15] (on the basis of electron microscope and X-ray diffraction evidence) explains these changes in terms of filament interaction. According to this theory, when a muscle contracts, the thick and thin filaments retain their original length but slide past one another so that their degree of interdigitation increases. The thin filaments extend farther into the *A* band, thus decreasing the *H* band region and ultimately obliterating it. As a result of this, the thin filament penetration into the *A* band brings the *Z* bands closer to the ends of the *A* band and as the sliding occurs, the sarcomere length is decreased.

At a finer level of resolution the thicker filament is found to be composed of myosin molecules arranged so that the backbone of the filament is composed of the tails of the molecules and the heads project out to form cross bridges (see Fig. VII–4). These cross bridges are believed to be the part of the myosin molecule which contains ATPase activity and actin-binding ability.[19] Each thin filament consists of a double helix of actin monomer units (see Fig. VII–4). Additional proteins, including *troponin* and *tropomyosin*, appear to be associated with the actin filaments. The monomer units of actin have a molecular weight of about 60,000. The actin can form a complex with the myosin and hence establish tension during contraction, but troponin will prevent the formation of this complex as long as calcium ion is not present in sufficient concentration. The concentration of calcium ions varies with the stage of the contraction–relaxation cycle.

It is known that the entire muscle cell contracts in response to the arrival of a nerve impulse at the neuromuscular junction. The release of acetylcholine from synaptic vesicles within the nerve ending depolarizes the muscle cell membrane, as we shall describe below. This depolarization initiates an action potential that is propagated along the muscle cell membrane. The action potential arrives at the invaginating *T*-tubule membrane and is then propagated along the membrane of the *T*-tubule into the interior portion of the muscle cell where it triggers the release of calcium ions from closely associated membranes of the sarcoplasmic reticulum. Calcium ions bind to the troponin as the calcium ion concentration rises above $10^{-6}\,M$. The cross bridges can then become attached to the actin filaments. Tension is generated and the muscle cell begins to shorten. After the passage of the impulse, the sarcoplasmic reticulum removes calcium ions from solution by active transport and sequesters them. This causes the calcium ion concentration surrounding the myofibrils to fall beneath $10^{-7}\,M$.[19] When the calcium ion concentration is less than $10^{-7}\,M$, troponin once again prevents the binding of actin and myosin and the system no longer contracts. (For additional information, the following excellent reviews are available: refs. 6,14,18.)

Neurons and Their Contacts. From the foregoing discussion of photoreception and muscle contraction it should be evident that nerve impulses are responsible for eliciting and coordinating many functions in the living organism. The cells that respond to various stimuli and transmit impulses from one area of the body to another are called *neurons,* or nerve cells. A neuron consists of a cell body, the *perikaryon* (which contains the nucleus), and a number of extending cytoplasmic processes. Neurons usually have several short *dendrites,* which conduct impulses toward the perikaryon, and only one long *axon,* which conducts impulses away from the cell body. These nerve cells vary tremendously in shape, size, number of processes, and the degree to which their processes branch. It is through their specialized contacts with each other (synapses) and with other cell types (neuromuscular junctions) that neurons are able to coordinate and maintain the many functions of the body. For this reason we briefly focus our attention upon these cell-to-cell contact sites.

Synapses. As we have indicated, specialized contact areas exist between adjacent neurons as well as between nerve cells and receptors (rod cells) and nerve cells and effectors (skeletal muscle cells). The anatomical and functional contact sites between adjacent nerve cells are called *synapses.* The nerve terminal endings at synapses display a variety of different shapes and sizes. For example, such presynaptic terminals may assume the form of bulbs, buttons, clubs, or cups. Within the presynaptic terminal are mitochrondria and a number of synaptic vesicles. The vesicles tend to cluster close to localized densities existing along the presynaptic membrane. Biochemical studies on isolated synaptic vesicles reveal that they are sites where *neurotransmitters* are stored.[8] Neurotransmitters are chemical substances that alter the ionic permeability of the postsynaptic membrane, making it either more or less permeable to ions. The primary sympathetic nervous system neurotransmitter is *norepinephrine,* while *acetylcholine* serves this purpose in the parasympathetic nervous system. The arrival of the nerve impulse at the presynaptic terminal ending appears to cause the synaptic vesicles to release their neurotransmitter contents into the synaptic cleft (existing between the pre- and postsynaptic membranes). The neurotransmitter diffuses across the synaptic cleft and affects the ionic permeability of the postsynaptic membrane. When the postsynaptic membrane is made excitable, the nerve impulse is therefore transmitted across the synapse and is propagated along the next neuron in the chain. As a result of this mechanism, transmission across synapses is unidirectional. The transmission process continues until the terminal effector is reached.

Within the central nervous system (brain and spinal cord) there are a phenomenal number of synaptic contacts between neurons. For example, many thousands of terminal endings synapse upon the cell body of a single large motor neuron, whose long axon is destined to terminate in skeletal muscle. Some of these synapses are *excitatory* (have a tendency to discharge the large motor neuron), while others are *inhibitory* (they tend to decrease the excitability of the neuron). Inhibitory synapses make it more difficult for nerve impulses to be transmitted to particular neurons and thus play important roles in coordinating body activities.

Chemical synapses appear to be the most common functional contact for the transmission of nerve impulses, although electrical synapses also occur.[10,11] In contrast to chemical synapses, no delay is recorded as a nerve impulse is transmitted across electrical synapses. Electron microcopical observations of electrical synapses show that they are formed by a specialization of the outer leaflets of the pre- and postsynaptic membranes. When seen in surface views, the synaptic membranes display an hexagonal subunit pattern.[22] These synapses appear similar to certain gap junctions (discussed in Chapter IV) which also display an hexagonal subunit pattern.[21] This hexagonal specialization is thought to allow ionic communication and somehow permit the impulse to be conducted electrically from one cell to another (a phenomenon known as *electrical coupling*).

Neuromuscular Junctions. As indicated above, the *neuromuscular junction* (also called a *motor end plate)* is a region of specialization between the nerve cell *axon* terminal and the striated muscle cell membrane (Fig. VII–9). It is differentiated to facilitate transmission of an impulse. The naked axon terminal inhabits a depression in the surface of the striated muscle cell membrane. Invaginating into the muscle cell from this cupped indentation are deep junctional folds. The cup-shaped area between the naked axon terminal and the muscle cell, and the extracellular area bordered by the junctional folds form the *synaptic cleft.* The synaptic cleft is filled by a dense amorphous material. *Acetylcholinesterase* (the enzyme which inactivates acetylcholine) has been localized in this area by electron microscopical cytochemistry.[1]

The axon terminal contains many mitochondria and small vesicles. The vesicles are most abundant near the region of contact between the nerve and muscle and they are thought to contain the neurotransmitter substance *acetylcholine*.[8] The most widely accepted theory of chemical neurotransmission across the motor end plate is that the synaptic vesicles release their transmitter into the extracellular synaptic cleft. This release presumably causes a change in the permeability and electrical potential of the muscle cell membrane. The membrane therefore becomes depolarized, resulting in an action potential which is propagated along the cell and which serves as a signal for contraction.

REFERENCES

[1] R. J. Barrnett, "The Fine Structural Localization of Acetylcholinesterase at the Myoneural Junction," *J. Cell Biol.,* 12 (1962), 247–262.

[2] W. Beermann, "Cytological Aspects of Information Transfer in Cellular Differentiation," *Amer. Zool.,* 3 (1963), 23–32.

[3] William Bloom and D. W. Fawcett, *A Textbook of Histology,* 9th ed. (Philadelphia: W. B. Saunders Company, 1968).

[4] M. S. Bretscher, "How Repressor Molecules Function," *Nature,* 217 (1968), 509–511.

[5] Ulrich Clever, "Von der Ecdysonkonzentration abhängige Genaktivitätsmuster in den Speicheldrüsenchromosomen von *Chironomus tentans,*" *Dev. Biol.,* 6 (1963), 73–98.

[6] "Comparative Aspects of Muscle," Graham Hoyle, ed., *Amer. Zool.,* 7 (1967), 433–669.

[7] E. D. P. DeRobertis, "Electron Microscope Observations on the Submicroscopic Organization of the Retinal Rods," *J. Biophys. Biochem. Cytol.,* 2 (1956), 319–330.

[8] E. D. P. DeRobertis, *Histophysiology of Synapses and Neurosecretion* (New York: Pergamon Press, Inc., 1964).

[9] J. D. Ebert, *Interacting Systems in Development* (New York: Holt, Rinehart and Winston, Inc., 1965).

[10] E. J. Furshpan and D. D. Potter, "Mechanism of Nerve-Impuse Transmission at a Crayfish Synapse," *Nature,* 180 (1957), 342–343.

[11] Kiyoshi Hama, "Some Observations on the Fine Structure of the Giant Fibers of the Crayfishes (*Cambarus virilus* and *Cambarus clarkii*) with Special Reference to the Submicroscopic Organization of the Synapses," *Anat. Rec.,* 141 (1961), 275–293.

[12] Jean Hanson and H. E. Huxley, "The Structural Basis of Contraction in Striated Muscle," in *Fibrous Proteins and Their Biological Significance,* Symp. Soc. Exp. Biol. No. IX (New York: Cambridge University Press, 1955), 228–264.

[13] Henry Harris, *Nucleus and Cytoplasm* (New York: Oxford University Press, Inc., 1968).

[14] H. E. Huxley, "The Fine Structure of Striated Muscle and Its Functional Significance," in *The Harvey Lectures,* Ser. 60 (New York: Academic Press Inc., 1966), 85–118.

[15] A. F. Huxley and R. Niedergerke, "Structural Changes in Muscle during Contraction," *Nature,* 173 (1954), 971–973.

[16] Francois Jacob and Jacques Monod, "Genetic Regulatory Mechanisms in the Synthesis of Proteins," *J. Mol. Biol.,* 3 (1961), 318–356.

[17] M. M. K. Nass, "Mitochondrial DNA: Advances, Problems and Goals," *Science,* 165 (1969), 25–35.

[18] L. D. Peachey, "Muscle," *Ann. Rev. Physiol.,* 30 (1968), 401–440.

[19] S. V. Perry, "Introduction to: Contractile Processes in Striated Muscle," in *The Contractile Process* (Boston: Little, Brown and Co., 1967), 63–70.

[20] K. R. Porter and Clara Franzini-Armstrong, "The Sarcoplasmic Reticulum," *Sci. Amer.,* 212 (1965), 72–80.

[21] J. P. Revel and M. J. Karnovsky, "Hexagonal Array of Subunits in Intercellular Junctions of the Mouse Heart and Liver," *J. Cell Biol.,* 33 (1967), C7–C12.

[22] J. D. Robertson, "The Occurrence of a Subunit Pattern in the Unit Membranes of Club Endings in Mauthner Cell Synapses in Goldfish Brains," *J. Cell Biol.,* 19 (1963), 201–221.

[23] F. S. Sjöstrand, "Electron Microscopy of the Retina," in *The Structure of the Eye*, Vol. 1, G. K. Smelzer, ed. (New York: Academic Press Inc., 1961), 1–28.

[24] T. M. Sonneborn, "Does Preformed Cell Structure Play an Essential Role in Cell Heredity?" in *The Nature of Biological Diversity*, J. M. Allen, ed. (New York: McGraw-Hill, 1963), 165–221.

[25] Curt Stern, "Two or Three Bristles," *Amer. Sci.*, 42 (1954), 213–247.

[26] George Wald, "The Molecular Organization of Visual Systems," in *Light and Life*, W. D. McElroy and Bentley Glass, eds. (Baltimore: Johns Hopkins Press, 1961), 724–753.

VIII

HOW TISSUES TRANSPORT SUBSTANCES

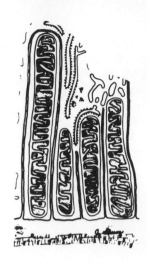

All cells can take in certain substances and rid themselves of others. Certain cells are capable of taking up a substance at one of their surfaces, transferring it through their cytoplasm, and releasing it from another surface. This entire process is called transcellular transport. In some cases the movement of a substance through the cell occurs without the utilization of energy, while in other cases cellular energy must be expended in order to accomplish the movement of a particular substance. This chapter discusses the transcellular transport of a variety of materials across two kinds of layers: endothelium and epithelium. Both of these layers are highly specialized, but in different ways, for cellular transport.

Endothelial cells line the lumen of all the blood vessels in the circulatory system, including the small capillaries where exchange between tissue and blood occurs. It is through this endothelial layer that nutrients, oxygen, waste products, and a variety of other substances that help to maintain the internal milieu of the body must pass. Endothelial cells are characterized by a thin layer of cytoplasm that contains few organelles.

Capillaries vary in their structure depending upon the particular tissue in which they are located. They may be classified by the kind of endothelium they possess.[22] Capillaries with a "continuous" endothelium exist in the lung, heart, skeletal muscle, and nervous system (Fig. VIII–1).[17] The endothelium in *continuous capillaries* forms a sheet of attached cells across which substances must be transported. These flat cells are about 0.1 to 0.5 micron thick, except in the area of their nucleus, where they bulge to a thickness of 1 to 5 microns.[17] The cytoplasm of these endothelial cells contains many micropinocytotic vesicles, 500 to 800 Ångström units in diameter.

Fenestrated capillaries exist in endocrine glands, the gastrointestinal tract, and the kidney (Fig. VIII–2). These vessels are ensheathed by a continuous basement membrane but their endothelial cells have fenestrae, or pores. These pores often are bridged by a thin layer of material (a diaphragm). When seen in surface view, the central area of the diaphragm exhibits increased density (Fig. VIII–3). Capillaries having this structure are very permeable to large molecules and their fenestrated endothelial cells are held accountable for this increased permeability. Again the structure of the cells is important in facilitating the rapid passage of large molecules.

Discontinuous capillaries, or *sinusoids,* exist in the liver, spleen, bone marrow, and in some other organs of the body. They do not have a continuous basement membrane and their endothelial cells are separated by large gaps. These "vessels" are extremely permeable, and leaky, as would be expected from their loosely organized structure.[20]

The main function of this thin endothelial layer is to retain large materials, such as red blood cells, in the plasma while facilitating the exchange of smaller molecules. It appears that much of the exchange of materials that occurs across endothelium does not involve an expenditure of energy by these lining cells.

Some epithelial cells constitute a second type of cellular layer, highly specialized for ion transport. These epithelial cells comprise an important part of a variety of organs and tissues such as the kidney and intestine, which are specialized for ion transport. In contrast to the exchange of materials by endothelial cells, the movement of ions by these ion-transporting cells requires large amounts of energy. To provide the needed energy for active transport, the epithelial cells contain many mitochondria (Fig. VIII–4). Generally speaking, the substances which are actively transported by cells are specific. (In this chapter we do not deal with the uptake of substances which undergo intracellular alteration. See Chapter VI for a discussion of this subject.)

TRANSPORT ACROSS CAPILLARY ENDOTHELIUM

Physiologists have learned much about the transport which occurs across the endothelium of capillaries.[33] The type of capillaries that have been most frequently studied has a continuous endothelium, which is not penetrated by pores. Three main types of transport processes occur which are characterized by the type of molecules involved. The first type of transport (type I) involves the passage of molecules which are soluble in lipids. For example, oxygen and carbon dioxide are lipid-soluble molecules. The second type of transport (type II) involves the passage of small lipid-insoluble molecules and water. Examples of lipid-insoluble molecules are sodium ions and chloride ions. The third type of transport (type III) concerns the passage of extremely large molecules such as large proteins.

Type I Transport. The transcapillary transport of oxygen and carbon dioxide (type I), both of which are lipid soluble, occurs at a rapid rate. Renkin [35] studied certain substances to determine the relationship between their capillary permeability and lipid solubility. He showed that compounds like glycerol and its derivatives rapidly passed through capillary walls. The rate of passage of these substances occurred in relation to their lipid solubility. The more lipid soluble the substance, the more rapid its rate of passage. This is consistent with lipid-soluble molecules penetrating directly through the lipid areas of the membrane. It is known that the rate of transport of lipid-soluble substances is many times greater than the rate for lipid-insoluble molecules of the same size. This indicates that lipid-soluble substances can penetrate larger areas of the capillary wall than are available to lipid-insoluble molecules. Since the permeability characteristics demonstrated in this type of transport are similar to those known to exist across cell membranes in general (see Chapter III), for transcapillary transport to occur these substances appear to penetrate directly both the luminal and basal membranes of the endothelial cell. However, morphological evidence for the pathway involved in this type of transport is lacking, because as yet no method exists whereby any of these small molecules can be visualized during their passage across the capillary endothelium.

Type II Transport. Pappenheimer's classic study [33] presents a transport route which takes into account the measured rates of passage of lipid-insoluble molecules and water across endothelium (type II). He postulated that the endothelium could have water-filled cylindrical channels or pores through which the substances moved. The total cross-sectional area of the pores could comprise less than 0.2 percent of the histological surface of the capillaries. [33] Pappenheimer calculated that uniform cylindrical pores with a diameter of 30 to 45 Ångström units and a population density of 1 to 2×10^9 per square centimeter of capillary wall would account for the observed rate of movement of lipid-insoluble molecules. Although he based his calculations on cylindrical pores, he saw no reason why the pores could not be another shape. He suggested that they might even, for example, be slits (intercellular channels) limited to the areas between the cells. *Diffusion* is probably responsible for much of the net movement of lipid-insoluble molecules through the pores. If the net movement resulted only from volume flow, the transport process would be extremely slow, whereas in reality the process is rapid. However, in reality the diffusion is probably restricted. If totally free diffusion occurred, water, sodium chloride, urea, and glucose could move through the capillary wall in both directions at rates estimated to be respectively 80, 40, 30, and 10 times faster than the rate at which these substances are, in fact, brought to the tissue by the incoming blood. Although the measured diffusion rates are rapid for small molecules, they are not as rapid as they would be if free diffusion were operating. Therefore, the concept of *restricted diffusion* has been developed to account for this slower rate of transport. Restricted diffusion also explains *molecular sieving*, which is the progressive decrease in apparent pore area available as the molecular size of the transported molecule increases. There is less restriction of small molecules to diffusion, but as molecules increase in size, their restriction to diffusion become much greater. This so-called molecular sieving would be seen if diffusion were occurring through pores with a small diameter.[33]

What is the morphological counterpart of the small-pore system? Cylindrical pores with a diameter in the range of 30 to 45 Ångström units might be visible in electron micrographs of capillary endothelium if they are present. However, such pores have not been observed.[2,3,16] Electron micrographs of capillaries in muscle tissue (i.e., the kind of tissue used for the physiological measurements just described) show that the capillary endothelium is composed of one single thin layer of endothelial cells resting upon a thin basement membrane (Fig. VIII–3). These cells are joined to their neighbors by specialized attachment sites. Along both the luminal and basal surfaces of the capillary endothelium, little cave-like structures (caveolae) can be seen.[32] Vesicular profiles of similar sizes and shapes are found near both surfaces and within the interior of the cell. The vesicles and caveolae have been thought to serve in the vesicular transport of material from one cell surface to the other.[30,31] The little cave-like structures at one surface of the cell might become filled with a substance to be transported. It could then pinch off to form a vesicle that would move across the cell and fuse with the cell membrane on the opposite surface, thus freeing the contents of the vesicles.

Could these entities be the morphological counterpart of the small-pore system? Problems arise in trying to equate vesicular transport with the data used to calculate pore size. For example, a vesicular transport mechanism of this nature does not explain the restricted diffusion and molecular sieving which has been measured in transport through capillaries of this type. Tracer substances, such as ferritin, can be used to trace the path of particle movement. When ferritin is injected into capillaries, the noted rate of vesicular transport is much too slow to account for the normal amount of water, ions, and other lipid-insoluble molecules transported.[16] Some physiologists have demonstrated that the diffusion of lipid-insoluble (type II) molecules is a passive process. This is incompatible with an energy-requiring vesicular transport mechanism.[16] The walls of these little caves show a positive reaction for the presence of an enzyme which splits nucleotide substrates such as ATP, indicating that the vesicular transport mechanism might, in fact, utilize ATP as an energy source.[23]

Caveolae and vesicles therefore appear as unlikely candidates for the morphological counterpart of the small-pore system proposed by the physiologists. Recent work[16] has revived the theory that the intercellular clefts between endothelial cells are the morphological equivalent of the small-pore system involved in transport of small lipid-insoluble substances. Horseradish peroxidase, which has a molecular weight of 40,000, has been used as a tracer for this class of substances. If horseradish peroxidase is injected intravenously, it becomes localized in the intercellular clefts between endothelial cells (Fig. VIII–5).[16] Horseradish peroxidase is the first tracer that has been seen in this position. Previous tracers (used as markers to follow the mechanism of transport in capillaries) have been much larger molecules with higher molecular weights and therefore could not serve to locate apparent sites for the transport of small lipid-insoluble molecules. Certain colloidal particles such as neutral lanthanum, when placed in the fixative solution, can also be seen in electron micrographs to gain access to the intercellular clefts.[16]

Careful study of electron micrographs taken from serial sections of capillaries indicate that in certain organs not all regions along the luminal border of the capillary are sealed by tight junctions. In one study, narrow gaps of approximately 40 Ångström units in capillaries of certain skeletal muscles were frequently found separating the two leaflets of the opposing cell membranes.[16] Other investigators have reported the presence of fused tight junctions between endothelial cells and did not report the presence of gaps.[28] However, these investigations were conducted primarily upon capillaries from the brain, which may be structurally different from muscle capillaries. Certainly brain capillaries demonstrate a decreased permeability to many substances. This decreased permeability in brain capillaries is known as the blood-brain barrier. However, other authors found fused tight junctions, effectively sealing off the intercellular clefts, in tissues similar to those used for the study of the horseradish peroxidase transport.[2,3] The reasons for these conflicting results have not been found.

If the intercellular clefts are the morphological counterpart for the small pore, thepassage of material through them could explain the restriction to diffusion and molecular sieving which were measured in experiments using capillary endothelium from muscle tissue. The passage of material through the intercellular clefts would presumably be a passive process. The forces which cause this type of transport would be diffusion and filtration, which in fact correlates with the physiological studies on the movement of lipid-insoluble molecules.

The surface area calculated by the physiologists to be necessary for the transport of lipid-insoluble molecules is much larger[33] than the surface area occupied by the intercellular clefts.[16] The effective path length (the length of the narrow cleft passage way), however, appears to be in the order of 100 to 400 Ångström units[16] and not as long as the figure used by physiologists (10^{-4} cm or 10,000 Ångström units) for their calculations of pore area.[33] If the effective path length (or narrow zone) is actually much shorter than the figure used in the original calculation, the discrepancy between the surface area as calculated by the physiologists, and that measured in electron micrographs of intercellular clefts, could be explained.[16]

Type III Transport. A third type of transport (type III) dealing with large molecules also occurs through the walls of capillaries.[15,25,36] Although small proteins apparently are transported in a manner consistent with the pore concept just discussed, extremely large proteins do not seem to be handled in the same manner.

It should be expected that the ratio of the concentration of small proteins in lymph to that in plasma decreases with increasing molecular size. This is to be expected because of the difficulty which larger proteins experience in diffusion through capillary pores. However, this decrease is noted only with small proteins, and above a certain size no further decrease is seen. To explain this observation, some physiologists[15,25] have proposed that a second system of pores is operating in addition to the small pore system already discussed. This system may be a less extensive one, having large openings or leaks. On the other hand it could involve transport by means of vesicle movement. Such a transport mechanism would presumably function to distribute large protein molecules such as antibodies and large hormones.

A large protein can be given intravenously to an animal and its location in the capillary wall can be observed in the electron microscope. This technique tests for type III transport mechanism by showing the site of transport of the large protein. When this experiment is done using the protein ferritin, the vesicles and caveolae of the endothelium are found to contain ferritin particles.[2,3,30,31,32] The time course of this type of transport has been determined in a recent study utilizing capillaries from rat diaphragm muscle.[3] Two minutes after the injection of ferritin, the tracer is found in the blood plasma and in vesicles on the luminal surface of the endothelium. After 10 minutes a small number of ferritin molecules can be seen in the connective tissue bordering the basal surface of the endothelium. By 1 hour many particles are found in the connective tissue and some appear in macrophages located along the basal surfaces. At 1 day the number of particles seen in the connective tissue approaches the number originally seen in the blood plasma, and by 4 days all particles appear to have been cleared from the blood and the endothelium. Particles of ferritin were not seen in cell junctions, intercellular clefts, or in the cytoplasmic matrix of the cells. Therefore, it may be concluded that in muscle capillaries these vesicles are the structural equivalent of the large-pore system proposed by physiologists. Additional studies are needed before these results on rat diaphragm muscle capillaries[3] can be generalized even to other capillaries which have the same appearance in electron micrographs. Physiological studies have repeatedly demonstrated that capillaries do differ with respect to their function,[33] and additional investigations of specialized capillaries, such as those found in the brain, still must be undertaken.

Fenestrated Capillaries and Filtration at the Renal Corpuscle. Muscle capillaries have been the type most thoroughly studied by both physiologists and anatomists, but other types of capillaries also exist in the body. For example, in the gastrointestinal mucosa a fenestrated capillary occurs. Its endothelial wall is much thinner and frequently penetrated by a system of pores approximately 350 to 450 Ångström units in diameter. In electron micrographs, these pores are often seen to be bridged by a thin *diaphragm*. Physiologists have shown that permeability of this type of capillary is greater than the permeability measured in muscle capillaries.[33] When horseradish peroxidase and ferritin are used as tracers for the small and large pores, respectively, in this fenestrated type of capillary from the intestine, both pore systems appear to be located in the fenestrae.[6] The horseradish peroxidase appears to traverse all of the fenestrated apertures. The ferritin appears to pass through only a few of the fenestrae. These fenestrae may lack part or all of the diaphragm material.[6]

The renal corpuscle contains an extensive capillary network gloved by a layer of epithelial cells (Fig. VIII–6). In the renal corpuscle, the hydrostatic pressure of the blood causes a portion of the plasma to be filtered out of the capillaries and across the layer of epithelial cells. In order to allow filtration to occur, the cells of both the capillaries and the epithelial coat are specialized. The basement membrane between the endothelial and epithelial cell layers of the renal corpuscle is a gel-like substance also permitting fluid to be filtered. The epithelial cells are like octopi with numerous long processes. These long processes in turn have numerous smaller processes or feet. A vast interdigitation of these small foot-like processes occurs, forming numerous intercellular channels bridged by a membrane (the filtration slit membrane). The filtration barrier of the renal corpuscle therefore has three components: the endothelial pore, the basement membrane, and the channels between the epithelial cells (Fig. VIII–7).

ION-TRANSPORTING TISSUES

There is another type of epithelium which is specialized to transport material in quite a different manner. In this epithelium, specific ions such as sodium are moved across cell layers and cellular energy is required for the process. The ability to actively move certain ions across a single cell membrane is a property of almost all cells. In general, it serves to oppose the passive influx of ions such as sodium. If active transport is inhibited, water accompanies the influx of sodium ions and the cell will swell until it bursts.

During the course of evolution, certain cells have become polarized. That is, they have developed the ability to handle ions differently at their various surfaces and as a result can move ions across themselves. This ability of certain epithelia to selectively move ions across themselves has been utilized for osmoregulation by animals living under various external conditions. Such epithelia are found in a number of species and in a variety of tissue. Examples of such epithelia are cells of the renal nephron, intestine, gall bladder, amphibian skin, amphibian bladder, and other specialized salt-transporting epithelia such as the nasal glands of birds and the rectal gland of dogfish. How these specialized cells handle the same three groups of substances follows.

Type I Transport. Oxygen, carbon dioxide, and small lipid-soluble molecules (type I) presumably move through the cell membrane into the cell in a manner similar to that occurring at both surfaces of the endothelial cell. They do not appear to be transported transcellularly in this tissue but instead are utilized or produced by the epithelial cells.

Type II Transport. Specific ions such as sodium appear to be moved across this kind of epithelium by a process which requires cell energy and is therefore called *active transport*. Other ions such as chloride, as well as water, appear to follow passively because of electrochemical or osmotic gradients set up by the active transport of the specific ions. Our attention is focused upon the active transport of sodium ions as an example of active transcellular transport. It appears that sodium is the ion most frequently transported, and the mechanisms involved in its movement have been extensively studied by many scientists. Also, sodium ions are worthy of detailed examination because of their great importance as a major extracellular electrolyte in a wide variety of organisms. In fact, all cells seem to be able to actively remove sodium ions from their intracellular environment, an ability which appears to be necessary to animal cells in order for them to maintain osmotic equilibrium. Many tissues, however, not only have the ability to move sodium out of cells, but by the transcellular transport of sodium ions can move sodium across an entire cell layer. They do this by extruding sodium ions actively only at certain surfaces. This mechanism of active sodium transport serves a number of important functions. For example, the cells of the nasal glands of marine birds excrete excess sodium chloride from the body, thus allowing the birds to survive in a marine environment. These birds drink only sea water and eat food having a high salt content, and it is essential to their survival that excess salt be eliminated. Transcellular movement of sodium ions is also a necessary function of the mammalian kidney. For example, in man, approximately 180 liters of fluid are filtered into the nephrons each day. Unless the nephrons return much of the filtered sodium ions and water back into the blood, extensive salt and water loss, and possibly even death, results.

Criteria have been established to determine whether or not a substance is actively transported by a cell. If the substance is able to move against an electrochemical gradient, it is generally thought to be actively transported. In order to determine if there is an electrochemical gradient, it is necessary to measure the concentration of the substance at both surfaces of the transporting cell membrane, and to know the *potential differences* across the surface of the membrane. It is then possible to calculate whether the movement of a specific substance at that site is against an electrochemical gradient. If a negative gradient does exist, the substance is actively transported. However, certain other features, such as solvent drag and the presence of substances which facilitate diffusion (permeases), must also be taken into consideration. When distal tubular cells of the kidney in the urodele *Necturus* were studied, active transport of sodium ion was localized in the basal region of the cells.[24] Located in this region of kidney tubule cells from a variety of species (Fig. VIII–8) is an extensive system of interdigitating lateral cell processes extending from adjacent cells. Within these lateral cytoplasmic processes, many mitochondria exist in close association with the lateral cell membranes. An enzyme having the ability to split ATP has been localized to the lateral cell membranes in a variety of ion-transporting tissues such as kidney, gall bladder,[18] and frog skin.[13] Such experimental data suggest that these lateral cell membranes are frequently sites of active sodium ion transport.

The transcellular transport of sodium ions in tissue such as kidney is thought to involve the following steps. Sodium ions supposedly migrate passively through the apical cell membrane. They are then able to diffuse through a portion of the cytoplasm and can be actively extruded into the lateral intercellular spaces by the enzyme systems of the lateral cell membranes. Most epithelia involved in the active movement of sodium ions are only one cell thick. However, this is not always the case. For example, frog skin is an epithelium that is several cell layers thick. It is well known that this tissue has the ability to actively transport sodium ions across its many cell layers. In frog skin ATPase activity has been demonstrated on the lateral cell surfaces of all cell layers, but it has not been observed on the basal cell surfaces.[13] Therefore, in frog skin sodium ions presumably migrate through the apical cell membranes of the top layer and from there they can move laterally from cell to cell at specialized sites within the epithelium. These sites of low electrical resistance have been shown to exist in normal epithelial layers from a number of animals and may serve as the means by which ions move from one cell to another.[5] The sodium ions make their way into any of the cell layers and then may be actively transported laterally into the intercellular spaces.

The steps of the process by which cells accomplish the movement of sodium ions have been studied by a number of investigators.[37] Many characteristics and aspects of the process have been identified and they include the following: (1) active transport has been shown to be driven by energy in the form of ATP; (2) the isolation of a Na^+-K^+ activated enzyme system has been accomplished and this system appears to be involved in active sodium transport; (3) this enzyme system has two separate sites, one with an affinity for Na^+ and another for K^+, which may serve as carrier sites for ion transport; (4) there are changes in the affinity for ions at these two sites which appear to be related to the presence of ATP, so it is likely that this enzyme system is the transport system; (5) the hydrolysis of ATP leads to phosphorylation of a compound in the enzyme system.

The model below was proposed by Skou[37] and indicates one possible explanation of how a sodium ion can be actively moved through a cell membrane in exchange for a potassium ion moved in the opposite direction. In step I, the transport system is postulated to have an inner and an outer surface. In this nonactivated state, sodium ions have an affinity for the outer surface and potassium ions have an affinity for the inner surface. Presumably the transport system can react with magnesium ions and ATP forming the activated compound seen in step II. This activation leads to a change in the affinity for sodium ions and potassium ions. Therefore, on the outer surface sodium ions move into the interstitial fluid in exchange for potassium ions which become bound to the active site. On the inner surface, the opposite occurs as potassium ions are released into the cell and sodium ions appear to be more closely bound to the active enzyme site. When potassium ions are on the outer site o, ATP can be hydrolyzed. This ATP hydrolysis causes deactivation of the transport system and some change occurs in the transport system

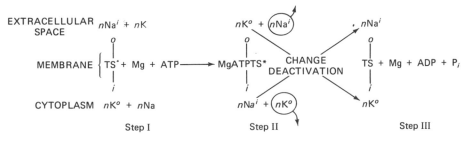

$$TS = \text{transport system}$$
$$i = \text{inside membrane}$$
$$o = \text{outside membrane}$$

so that the sodium and potassium ions exchange positions. How the sodium and potassium ions exchange positions as the result of deactivation of the transport system is not completely understood. Perhaps this change results from some reversible effect on the structure of the enzyme system. A new active transport process, or ATP cycle, can then begin as the transport system again reacts with magnesium ions and ATP. In this model transport system, sodium ions have moved from the inside of the cell to the outside, and potassium ions have moved in the opposite direction.

The active transcellular transport of sodium ions is frequently accompanied by a passive movement of chloride ions because of the resulting electrochemical gradient. It is also accompanied by a passive transport of water which accompanies the process because of osmotic pressure gradients.

Serial Membrane Model. In studies with rat intestine, an apparent contradiction of this osmotic water movement has been observed. Water movement from mucosal (luminal surface) to serosal surface occurred even though the solute concentration was higher on the mucosal surface. Therefore, water appeared to be moving from a lower to a higher chemical potential (against osmosis).[34] In addition, in hamster intestine it was noted that a small hydrostatic pressure applied to the serosal surface of the intestine stopped this net water transport.[38] To explain what appeared to be water moving from a lower to a higher chemical potential in this system, Curran and associates[7,8,9,29] proposed a model depicting water transport coupled to active ion transport in this system. This model is called the *serial membrane model* (Fig. VIII–9). Consider a closed system constituted by compartments *A, B,* and *C.* Between *A* and *B* is a thin membrane (1) having small pores. Between *B* and *C* is a thick membrane

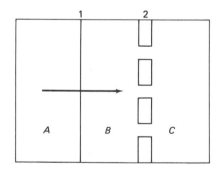

FIGURE VIII–9. Diagram of the serial membrane model showing a closed system with compartments *A, B,* and *C.* Between *A* and *B* is a thin membrane having small pores. Between *B* and *C* is a thick membrane with large pores. Modified from Peter Curran, *Fed. Proc.*, 24 (1965), 993.

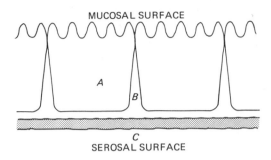

FIGURE VIII–10. Diagram showing postulated cellular counterparts for compartments *A*, *B*, and *C*.

(2) with large pores. Assume that active transport of a solute can occur from *A* to *B* across the thin membrane. After active transport of the solute, the concentration of solute will be higher in *B* than in any other compartment. Therefore, water moves passively from *A* into *B*. This movement of water increases the hydrostatic pressure in compartment *B*. The increase in hydrostatic pressure drives fluid through the larger pores of membrane 2 into compartment *C*. This passive movement of fluid, coupled to active sodium transport, is consistent with the measurements obtained in studies of active transport in intestine. In cell systems (Fig. VIII–10), compartment *A* is equivalent to the cytoplasm of the cell, compartment *B* corresponds to the intercellular space, and compartment *C* corresponds to the connective tissue beneath the basement membrane. The active driving force for the system is the lateral cell membrane between compartments *A* and *B*.

The serial membrane model has also been used to explain active sodium transport in the gall bladder where large spaces develop intercellularly during the active solute transport.[18] This kind of transport mechanism could also be operative in tissues which do not show a large increase in their intercellular spaces. In fact, this mechanism would be more efficient in such cases because if the lateral intercellular volume does not increase, a given amount of water would cause a greater increase in hydrostatic pressure. An example of a tissue which may operate in such a manner is the proximal tubule of the mammalian kidney.

The serial membrane model may also serve to explain ion movement in tissues where sodium ions move in the opposite direction, that is, from the serosal to the mucosal surface.[10] This kind of transport appears to occur within the rectal gland of the dogfish, the nasal glands of birds, and the Malpighian tubules of insects. In such cases, active solute transport would occur from *B* to *A* coupled with water transport in that same direction. The result would be a decrease in hydrostatic pressure in compartment *B* causing the subsequent movement of water from *C* to *B*

Because the lateral cell membrane is the site of the motive forces, an increase in its surface area should increase the area involved in coupled transport. It is a well-known fact that tissue highly specialized for actively transporting ions, such as dogfish rectal gland, nasal glands of birds, and kidneys, have many lateral interdigitating cell processes. These processes increase the area of lateral cell membrane and presumably, therefore, the area of active ion transport. Mitochondria, which provide energy for this process, are seen closely associated with these lateral cell membranes (Fig. VIII–8).

Type III Transport. Does transcellular transport of large proteins or other large molecules (type III transport) also occur across epithelial layers? In studies where large protein molecules have been introduced into animals, the proteins appear to be picked up by endocytosis. They then appear to move inexorably into the lysosomes where digestion presumably occurs. This has been shown to occur repeatedly with a variety of proteins in a number of different cell types. For example, when hemoglobin[11,12,26,27] or horseradish peroxidase[14] is injected into the blood stream, it subsequently reaches the kidney where it is filtered at the renal corpuscle into the lumen of the nephron. The cells of the proximal convoluted tubule of the nephron will then take up the protein from the tubular lumen and it becomes sequestered within lysosomes. Subsequent digestion of the material by lysosomal enzymes appears to result (see Chapter VI). It is not yet known whether or not epithelial cell layers can distinguish between various proteins, or whether different proteins are handled in particular ways. Repeated experimental studies have shown that most proteins and tracers taken up by the cells are sequestered into lysosomal compartments and digested. No experimental evidence is available to indicate that material can leave the lysosomal compartments and move across the cell.

There are hints, however, that another mechanism may exist. For example, in certain species, antibodies appear to pass through the intestinal epithelium for a short time after birth.[1] One study has reported that intact ferritin particles moved through cells and into the lateral intercellular spaces.[19]

A similar transport of large intact molecules has been proposed to occur in flounder kidney tubules.[21] If lysozyme (a small protein having a molecular weight of 14,000) is given to flounders, and the kidney tubules are subsequently isolated and incubated, 100 percent recovery of intact lysozyme protein is found possible.[21] If ferritin or other colloidal particles are injected retrograde into the nephrons of intact flounder kidneys, these particles are taken up and subsequently transported across the apical cell cytoplasm and into the lateral intercellular spaces (Fig. VIII–11).[4] Therefore, it appears that at least in this one cell type, large proteins have escaped the inevitable movement into the lysosomal compartments of the cell. Hence, it is conceivable that a type III transport of large molecules does exist for certain epithelial layers.

REFERENCES

[1] F. W. R. Brambell, "The Transmission of Immunity from Mother to Young and the Catabolism of Immunoglobulins," *Lancet,* 2 (1966), 1087–1093.

[2] R. R. Bruns and G. E. Palade, "Studies on Blood Capillaries. I. General Organization of Blood Capillaries in Muscle," *J. Cell Biol.,* 37 (1968), 244–276.

[3] R. R. Bruns and G. E. Palade, "Studies on Blood Capillaries. II. Transport of Ferritin Molecules across the Wall of Muscle Capillaries." *J. Cell Biol.,* 37 (1968), 277–299.

[4] R. E. Bulger and B. F. Trump, "A Mechanism for Rapid Transport of Colloidal Particles by Flounder Renal Epithelium," *J. Morphol.,* 127 (1969), 205–224.

[5] Stanley Bullivant and W. R. Loewenstein, "Structure of Coupled and Uncoupled Cell Junctions," *J. Cell Biol.,* 37 (1968), 621–632.

[6] F. Clementi and G. E. Palade, "Intestinal Capillaries. I. Permeability to Peroxidase and Ferritin," *J. Cell Biol.,* 41 (1969), 33–58.

[7] P. F. Curran, "Ion Transport in Intestine and Its Coupling to Other Transport Processes," *Fed. Proc.,* 24 (1965), 993–999.

[8] P. F. Curran and J. R. MacIntosh, "A Model System for Biological Water Transport," *Nature,* 193 (1962), 347–348.

[9] P. F. Curran and A. K. Solomon, "Ion and Water Fluxes in the Ileum of Rats," *J. Gen. Physiol.,* 41 (1957), 143–168.

[10] J. M. Diamond and W. H. Bossert, "Functional Consequences of Ultrastructural Geometry in 'backwards' Fluid-Transporting Epithelia," *J. Cell Biol.,* 37 (1968), 694–702.

[11] J. L. E. Ericsson, "Absorption and Decomposition of Homologous Hemoglobin in Renal Proximal Tubular Cells. An Experimental Light and Electron Microscopic Study," *Acta Path. et Microbiol. Scandinav. Suppl.,* 168 (1964), 1–121.

[12] J. L. E. Ericsson, "Transport and Digestion of Hemoglobin in the Proximal Tubule. II. Electron Microscopy," *Lab. Invest.,* 14 (1965), 16–39.

[13] M. G. Farquhar and G. E. Palade, "Adenosine Triphosphatase Localization in Amphibian Epidermis," *J. Cell Biol.,* 30 (1966), 359–379.

[14] R. C. Graham, Jr., and M. J. Karnovsky, "The Early Stages of Absorption of Injected Horseradish Peroxidase in the Proximal Tubules of Mouse Kidney: Ultrastructural Cytochemistry by a New Technique," *J. Histochem. Cytochem.,* 14 (1966), 291–302.

[15] Gunnar Grotte, "Passage of Dextran Molecules Across the Blood-Lymph Barrier," *Acta Chir. Scand. Suppl.,* 211 (1965), 1–84.

[16] M. J. Karnovsky, "The Ultrastructural Basis of Capillary Permeability Studied with Peroxidase as a Tracer," *J. Cell Biol.,* 35 (1967), 213–236.

[17] M. J. Karnovsky, "The Ultrastructural Basis of Transcapillary Exchanges," *J. Gen. Physiol.,* 52 (1968), 64s–95s.

[18] G. I. Kaye, H. O. Wheeler, R. T. Whitlock, and Nathan Lane, "Fluid Transport in the Rabbit Gallbladder. A Combined Physiological and Electron Microscopic Study," *J. Cell Biol.,* 30 (1966), 237–268.

[19] J.-P. Kraehenbuhl, E. Gloor, and B. Blanc, "Résorption intestinale de la ferritine chez deux espéique animales aux possibilités d'absorption protéique néonatale différentes," *Z. Zellforsch.,* 76 (1967), 170–186.

[20] L. V. Leak and J. F. Burke, "Fine Structure of the Lymphatic Capillary and the Adjoining Connective Tissue Area," *Amer. J. Anat.,* 118 (1966), 785–809.

[21] Thomas Maack and W. B. Kinter, "Transport of a Small Molecular Weight Protein, Lysozyme, in Dissected and Incubated Tubular Masses of the Flounder Kidney," *Bull. Mt. Dessert Isl. Biol. Lab.,* 7 (1967), 27–29.

[22]G. Majno, "Ultrastructure of the Vascular Membrane," in *Handbook of Physiology,* Section 2: Circulation, W. F. Hamilton and Philip Dow, eds. (Washington, D.C., Amer. Physiological Society, 1965), Vol. III, 2293–2375.

[23]V. T. Marchesi and R. J. Barrnett, "The Demonstration of Enzymatic Activity in Pinocytic Vesicles of Blood Capillaries with the Electron Microscope," *J. Cell Biol.,* 17 (1963), 547–556.

[24]D. L. Maude, Isam Shehadeh, and A. K. Solomon, "Sodium and Water Transport in Single Perfused Distal Tubules of Necturus Kidney," *Amer. J. Physiol.,* 211 (1966), 1043–1049.

[25]H. S. Mayerson, C. G. Wolfram, H. H. Shirley, Jr., and K. Wasserman, "Regional Differences in Capillary Permeability," *Amer. J. Physiol.,* 198 (1960), 155–160.

[26]Fritz Miller, "Hemoglobin Absorption by the Cells of the Proximal Convoluted Tubule in Mouse Kidney," *J. Biophys. Biochem. Cytol.,* 8 (1960), 689–718.

[27]Fritz Miller and G. E. Palade, "Lytic Activities in Renal Protein Absorption Droplets. An Electron Microscopical Cytochemical Study," *J. Cell Biol.,* 23 (1964), 519–552.

[28]A. R. Muir and A. Peters, "Quintuple-Layered Membrane Junctions at Terminal Bars between Endothelial Cells," *J. Cell Biol.,* 12 (1962), 443–448.

[29]J. T. Ogilvie, J. R. McIntosh, and P. F. Curran, "Volume Flow in a Series-Membrane System," *Biochim. Biophys. Acta,* 66 (1963), 441–444.

[30]G. E. Palade, "Transport in Quanta Across the Endothelium of Blood Capillaries," *Anat. Rec.,* 136 (1960), 254.

[31]G. E. Palade, "Blood Capillaries of the Heart and Other Organs," *Circulation,* 24 (1961), 368–388.

[32]G. E. Palade and R. R. Bruns, "Structural Modulations of Plasmalemmal Vesicles," *J. Cell Biol.,* 37 (1968), 633–649.

[33]J. R. Pappenheimer, "Passage of Molecules through Capillary Walls," *Physiol. Reviews,* 33 (1953), 387–423.

[34]D. S. Parsons and D. L. Wingate, "Fluid Movements Across Wall of Rat Small Intestine in Vitro," *Biochim. Biophys. Acta,* 30 (1958), 666–667.

[35]E. M. Renkin, "Capillary Permeability to Lipid-Soluble Molecules," *Amer. J. Physiol.,* 168 (1952), 538–545.

[36]E. M. Renkin, "Transport of Large Molecules Across Capillary Walls," *The Physiologist,* 7 (1964), 13–28.

[37]J. C. Skou, "The Enzymatic Basis for the Active Transport of Sodium and Potassium," *Protoplasma,* 63 (1967), 303–308.

[38]T. H. Wilson, "A Modified Method for Study of Intestinal Absorption in Vitro," *J. Appl. Physiol.,* 9 (1956), 137–140.

SUMMARY

It is within its functioning cytoplasm that a cell expresses its individuality. Much remains to be learned about how these small units of life regulate and perform their amazing number of functions. With the advent of the electron microscope a new period of pure morphological description was begun. Today the electron microscope is becoming a tool to be used in conjunction with other biological techniques in an effort to learn more about normal and diseased cells.

The following is a brief recapitulation of some of the major functional processes of the cytoplasm as they are presently understood. The accompanying schematic drawing of a composite cell (Fig. S–1) identifies the pathways, and the various organelles, involved in these cellular functions. Certain features found only in specific cells are illustrated in this composite diagram.

Endocytosis is demonstrated in the upper left of the cell: (a) a particle becomes engulfed in an invagination of the cell membrane; (b) a vesicle buds off the plasma membrane, entrapping the particle; (c) fusion of several such vesicles forms a vacuole; (d) condensation of particulate matter occurs in the vacuole; (e) the condensed vacuole fuses with I° or II° lysosomes; (f) the lysosomal enzymes digest the material within the vacuole; (g) a residual body remains after digestion; (h) debris is excreted.

Autophagy is depicted in the upper central portion of the cell. An organelle, in this case a mitochondrion, becomes surrounded by smooth-surfaced membranes (i) which form a double-layered sac enclosing the organelle (j). The inner of the two membranes enclosing the organelle disappears leaving a single-membrane-limited inclusion body, the autophagic vacuole (k). Enzymatic digestion of the organelle, by lysosomal enzymes, leaves a residual body (1), which is released from the cell as debris by exocytosis.

Protein synthesis for secretion may occur via several routes (see arrows in the right upper portion of the cell). One route includes the following: ribosomes attached to the rough-surfaced endoplasmic reticulum synthesize proteins (m), which move into the cisternae of the endoplasmic riticulum. From the cisternae of the endoplasmic reticulum the protein enters the Golgi complex, presumably by budding from the rough-surfaced

119

endoplasmic reticulum to form vesicles, which then fuse with Golgi vacuoles (n). Progressive condensation (packaging) of the proteins occurs within the Golgi. The proteins are linked to carbohydrates forming glycoproteins within the final secretory granule (o). This pathway is also utilized for synthesizing mucopolysaccharides and lipoproteins which are destined for export. The granule moves apically (p) and its limiting membrane fuses with the surface cell membrane, releasing the protein contents to the exterior (q). In a second synthetic pathway, ribosomes on the outside of the rough-surfaced endoplasmic reticulum synthesize proteins which appear within nearby vesicles. The proteins then pass through condensing vacuoles (r) located near transitional elements of the Golgi complex. Progressive condensation leads to the formation of a granule (p), which moves apically in the cell, to await release. In some cells, for example fibroblasts, a route may exist whereby products synthesized by the rough-surfaced endoplasmic reticulum are excreted directly to the exterior of the cell. This would involve fusion of membranes derived from the endoplasmic reticulum cisternae with the surface cell membrane, and subsequent release of the contained products.

Cytoplasmic proteins are synthesized on polysomes free in the cytoplasm. Certain organelles, such as mitochondria and chloroplasts, appear to contain independent protein-synthetic systems capable of making some proteins needed in their construction.

The establishment of cell shape in differentiated cells is determined in part by microtubules (s) and microfilaments that can be organized into complex arrays for cell motility.

Transcellular ion transport is difficult to depict morphologically, but the enzymes responsible for this active transport mechanism are thought to reside in the lateral surface cell membranes. The cells of most tissues, which are highly specialized for transcellular transport of ions (such as kidney, and the nasal salt-excreting glands of marine birds), have increased their lateral surface areas by having many lateral or in some cases basal interdigitations (t). Mitochondria (u), which provide the necessary energy for the active transport process, lie very near these surface membranes. Transcellular transport involves the transfer of ions across cell layers and may be depicted according to the following steps: ions from a lumen move into the cell across its apical membrane and are actively transported across the lateral cell membrane into the intercellular compartment. From here they move basally in the extracellular space, thus completing their movement across a cell layer.

Ions can also move from cell to cell. In this case, they appear to traverse at specialized regions of cell-to-cell junctions. The gap junction is the best documented type of junction at which this appears to happen.

Much has been learned about the functioning cytoplasm—but much more remains to be learned.

INDEX